The Fas

Transfor

A Functional Guide to Burn Fat, Heal Your Body and Transform Your Life with Intermittent & Extended Fasting

Dr. David Jockers DNM, DC, MS

Michael Dugan BS, FDN-P

First published in 2020 by DrJockers.com

ISBN #: 979-8-561-99741-9

The information included in this book is for educational purposes only. It is not intended or implied to be a substitute for professional medical advice. The reader should always consult his or her healthcare provider to determine the appropriateness of the information for his or her own situation or if he or she has any questions regarding a medical condition or treatment plan. Reading the information in this book does not constitute a physician-patient relationship.

The statements in this book have not been evaluated by the Food and Drug Administration. The products or supplements in this book are not intended to diagnose, treat, cure or prevent any disease. The authors and publisher expressly disclaim responsibility for any adverse effects that may result from the use or application of the information contained in this book.

Cover and image design by Stephen Johnson

The Fasting Transformation:

Burn Fat, Heal Your Body & Transform Your Life

Our society is metabolically damaged, and this is causing us to be sick, fatigued and overweight. Our bodies should be powerful fat burners that create plenty of energy to keep us going all day long. Unfortunately, most people are settling for so much less than their best.

The answer to this comes down to an ancient healing strategy that optimizes nutrient timing to balance hormones and burn fat for fuel. This strategy cost nothing, is available to all and is quite simple to begin using.

Fasting is the most ancient, inexpensive and most powerful healing strategy known to mankind. All of our ancient ancestors practiced fasting in one way or the other and many great sages and cultures revered fasting for its physical, mental, emotional and spiritual benefits.

In this book, Dr. David Jockers takes you on a journey to help you understand the history and practical use for fasting to improve your life and health.

You will discover the science behind how fasting improves insulin sensitivity, hormone optimization, fat burning, stem cells and cellular healing. You will learn about how fasting holds promise for the prevention and treatment of major diseases such as cancer, autoimmune conditions, digestive disorders and neurodegenerative pathologies.

This book will go over all the various research and practical applications for daily intermittent fasting, partial fasting and extended fasting strategies. You will also learn how to troubleshoot challenges you may encounter on a fasting regimen.

This book is designed to help inspire and empower you to embrace a fasting lifestyle while enjoying tasty and healthy foods at the proper time to improve your metabolic flexibility and energy efficiency so you can burn fat for fuel and have all day energy.

Endorsements for This Book

Intermittent fasting is one of the best strategies to reset your metabolism, burn fat, improve your brain health and reduce your risk of chronic disease. Dr. David Jockers is one of the top thought leaders in this area and in this book, he will empower you on how to do this the right way.

He goes through how fasting can reduce your risk and even help you overcome cancer, autoimmune conditions, digestive challenges and neurodegenerative disease. You will also learn how to troubleshoot the challenges that come up and how to implement a lifestyle built around intermittent fasting! I highly recommend this book!

Dr. Josh Axe, DNM, DC, CNS
Founder of DrAxe.com and Ancient Nutrition
Author of *Eat Dirt*, *Keto Diet* and *The Collagen Diet*

As a cardiologist who practices naturally, I recommend intermittent fasting to all of my patients. And there is no better authority on fasting than my friend Dr. David Jockers. His new book is comprehensive and provides easy, actionable steps to fasting for heart health and so much more.

Dr. Jack Wolfson, DO, FACC
Author of *The Paleo Cardiologist*
Host of *The Healthy Heart Show* podcast

"The Fasting Transformation is a must read. As important as fasting is for our bodies, Dr. David Jockers will take you on a journey to understand why you must fast, and will help make it as healthy and easy for you as possible. I highly recommend this book."

Dr. Anna Cabeca, DO, FACOG
Best Selling Author of *The Hormone Fix* and *Keto-Green 16*

A lost healing art and regular spiritual practice since the dawn of humanity, everyone who is on a quest to enjoy the abundant life should be fasting in one form or another. In his brilliant book, Dr. Jockers takes out the guesswork and clearly lays the groundwork to help you tap into the true healing power of fasting with confidence and ease.

Dr. Eric Zielinski
Author of the National Bestseller *The Healing Power of Essential Oils*

I have taught fasting to doctors and health enthusiasts since the 1990's as a lost art to healing. Dr. David Jockers captures the art and science of fasting in such a simple and usable strategy to take your health to another level.

Fasting unlocks your genetic potential and is the oldest and most scientific key. We are all programmed in our DNA to fast for renewal and regeneration, and yet so few do it. If you desire to live long healthy start fasting now, and this book will act as the perfect guide.

Dr. Dan Pompa
Author of *Beyond Fasting*
Host of Cellular Healing TV

The new bible for intermittent and extended fasting. Dr. Jockers has done an amazing job breaking down the science of fasting, autophagy and the body's self-healing processes. His new book is a must read for anyone looking to attempt the intermittent and extended fasting in a safe and effective way. Highly recommended read!"

Dr. Peter Osborne D.PSc, DC, DACBN
International Best Selling Author of *No Grain No Pain*

Fasting is an ancient healing practice that supercharges the body to stimulate fat burning, reduce inflammation and prevent chronic disease. In this book, Dr. David Jockers does a great job of dispelling common myths involved with fasting while laying out the best strategies to support your body for success with intermittent fasting, partial fasting and extended fasting approaches.

Jordan Rubin
New York Times Bestselling Author of *The Maker's Diet*
Founder of Garden of Life and Ancient Nutrition

Fasting is an ancient healing practice that reduces inflammation, stimulates fat burning, activates autophagy and improves our cellular health. In this book, Dr. David Jockers shows you the best practices for incorporating intermittent fasting, partial and extended fasts.

He also goes deep into the research and shows you how fasting can help improve autoimmune conditions, neurological disorders and digestive ailments. I highly recommend this book to learn how to unlock your body's healing potential!!

Naomi Whittel
NY Times Best-Selling Author
Glow 15 and *High Fiber Keto*

Dr. David Jockers DNM, DC, MS

Dr. David Jockers is a doctor of natural medicine, who runs one of the most popular natural health websites in DrJockers.com which has gotten over 1 million monthly visitors and his work has been seen on popular media such as the Dr. Oz show and Hallmark Home and Family.

Dr. Jockers is the author of the best-selling book "The Keto Metabolic Breakthrough" by Victory Belt publishing and "The Fasting Transformation Summit." He is a world-renowned expert in the area of ketosis, fasting and functional nutrition. He is also the host of the Dr. Jockers Functional Nutrition podcast.

Dr. Jockers lives in Canton, Georgia with his wife Angel and his twin boys David & Joshua and his daughter Joyful.

Michael Dugan BS, FDN-P

Michael is a certified Functional Diagnostic Nutrition Practitioner and Human Biomechanics Specialist. He has worked with DrJockers.com doing research writing for the last 3 years.

Growing up as a competitive swimmer, ultimately becoming a Division-1 collegiate athlete, drove Michael to succeed, but also led to quite an extensive list of health challenges upon graduation. After resolving many mental and digestive issues through functional nutrition principles, he specialized in an often-undressed area of health - chronic pain.

Michael now focuses on resolution of chronic pain through functional movement with a heavy emphasis on a fasting-focused lifestyle. You can find his info at www.biomechanicsatlanta.com

Table of Contents

Introduction: The History of Fasting....6

History of Fasting....6

The Ancient Greeks....7

Fasting in Spiritual and Biblical Context....8

It's Time to Break the Societal Programming....10

Fasting is NOT Starvation....10

Past vs Current Uses for Fasting....11

Chapter 1: The Benefits of Fasting....13

Healing the Metabolism and Burning Fat....13

Restoring Insulin Sensitivity....14

Ultimate Anti-Inflammatory....15

Cellular Autophagy....16

Stem Cells....16

Youthful Hormones....18

Reduce Chronic Disease Risk....18

Improved Relationship with Food....19

Mental Health and Focus....20

Improved Energy....21

Healing the Digestive System....22

Heightened Intuition, Spiritual Guidance, Decision Making....23

The Global Metabolic Pandemic (and Why Everyone Should Consider Adopting a Fasting Lifestyle)....24

Chapter 2: The Science Behind Fasting....26

Fasting Mechanism: Insulin Sensitivity....27

Insulin Resistance....28

Symptoms of Insulin Resistance....28

How to Measure if You Are Insulin Resistant 29
Hemoglobin A1C (HbA1C) 29
Fasting Plasma Glucose Test (FPG) 30
Oral Glucose Tolerance Test (OGTT) 30
Continuous Blood Glucose Monitor 31
The Negative Feedback Loop of Energy Balance and Why Fasting is the Single Best Solution for Insulin Resistance 31
Here's What the Science Says........ 32
So, do these benefits apply to humans as well? 33

Fasting Mechanism: Ketosis 34

Benefits of Ketosis 34
Anti-Inflammatory 34
Improvement in Metabolic Conditions 35
Protection Against Neurodegenerative Diseases 35
Anxiolytic and Anti-Depressive Effects 36
Anti-Cancer & Chemotherapy Booster 36
Improvement in Mitochondrial Health 37

Fasting Mechanism: Increased Growth Hormone 38
Unfortunately, HGH levels tend to decline with age. 39
What Do You Do When HGH Plummets? 39
How Fasting Changes Growth Hormone 40

Fasting Mechanism: AMPk 41

Fasting Mechanism: Stem Cells 42

The Synergy of Benefits 44

Chapter 3: Fasting Myths........ 45

Fasting Myth: It is Unnatural and Unhealthy for the Body 45

Fasting Myth: It Slows Down Your Metabolism 46

Fasting Myth: It Causes Nutrient Deficiencies 47

Fasting Myth: It Causes Muscle Loss 48

Fasting Myth: Fasting is an Eating Disorder (Or Causes Them) 49

Fasting Myth: It is Dangerous for People with Diabetes 50
For Pre-Diabetics and Type 2 Diabetics 50
For Type I Diabetics 50

Fasting Myth: It Causes Binge Eating 51

Fasting Myth: You Shouldn't Exercise While Fasting 52

Fasting Myth: It Will Make You Feel Hangry 53

Fasting Myth: It Will Cause Food Cravings 54

Time to Implement! 54

Chapter 4: Intermittent Fasting Strategies **55**
Simple Fast 55
Brunch Fast 57
Crescendo Fast 57
Cycle Fast 59
Strong Fast 59
Warrior Fast and OMAD 61
Chapter 5: Weekly & Extended Fasting Strategies **62**
One Day a Week 62
5:2 Fasting 63
4:3 Fasting 64
Alternate-Day Fasting 65
Rolling 48-hour Fasts 66
Extended-Day Fasting 67
Chapter 6: Partial Fasting Strategies **69**
Bone Broth Fasting 70
Green Juice Fasting 74
Fasting Mimicking Diet 78
Implementing A Fasting Mimicking Diet 80
Fat or Keto Fast 82
Daniel Fast 84
Advantages of Partial Fasting Compared to Water Fasting 89
Downsides of Partial Fasting Compared to Water Fasting 90
Chapter 7: Fasting for Chronic Disease **91**
Cancer 91
Digestive Health 102
Autoimmune Disease 110
Neurodegeneration 115

Chapter 8: How to Begin Fasting 125

The Gradual and Comfortable Way 125

How to Know When You are Ready for the Next Step of Fasting 128

Fasting Strength Questionnaire 129

If You Are a Fasting Novice 131

If You Are a Fasting Pro 131

If You Are a Fasting Superhero 132

The Uncomfortable Way to Start Fasting: Extended Fasting 133

Chapter 9: What to Expect on a 5 Day Fast 135

Day 1 135

Day 1 Side Effects 136

Day 2 137

Day 2 Symptoms 138

Day 2 Health Effects 139

Day 3 140

Day 3 Health Effects 140

Gauging Your Day 3 Ketosis Adaptation 141

Day 4 142

Day 5 143

Breaking the Fast 144

How Often Should You Do an Extended Fast? 144

Chapter 10: Preparing for Your Extended Fast 146

Strategy #1: Reduce Your Schedule Demands 146

Strategy #2: GIVE YOURSELF PERMISSION TO REST 147

Strategy #3: Schedule a Spa Day 148

Strategy #4: Avoid People Who Will Not Support Your Efforts 149

Strategy #5: Drink Water 150

Strategy #6: Add Some Salt 151

Strategy #7: Get Sunshine & Ground Yourself 151
Strategy #8: Move, but Gently 152
Strategy #9: Use Natural Sweeteners If Needed 153
Strategy #10: Avoid the Kitchen the Best You Can 154

Chapter 11: Troubleshooting Fasting Challenges 155
Challenge #1: Dizziness, Fatigue, and Headaches 155
Challenge #2: Constipation 157
Challenge #3: Toxic Reactions 158
Challenge #4: Re-feeding Syndrome 160
Challenge #5: Feeling Cold 161
Supplements to Support Fasting 161
Will Taking Supplements Break a Fast? 162
Reasons to Supplement While Fasting 163

Chapter 12: The Fasting Lifestyle 171
So Let's Recap 171
The Most Important Benefits of Fasting That We've Uncovered Include: 172
Creating the Fasting Schedule That Fits your Needs 174
Importance of Feast-Famine Cycling 176
Thank You 177

References 178

Introduction: The History of Fasting

The Most Ancient, Inexpensive & Powerful Healing Strategy

If there was a free strategy, used by every renowned sage and spiritual leader throughout history, that could drastically improve your overall health and vitality – would you use it?

I think it is pretty reasonable to assume that most people would say "heck yes" to the question above. As you have already seen the title of this book (and likely bought it for that reason), you already know what this strategy is. Fasting.

Although fasting is one of the most powerful healing tools we have for health and performance, many people are still hesitant. Unaware of the rich history, scientific data, and anecdotal evidence that exists – many people believe fasting to be dangerous, unpleasant, or ineffective.

In this book, I will address and shed light on some of the most prominent concerns and dive deep into how fasting can be implemented for a variety of goals. As we progress through this book, I am going to uncover a brief history of fasting, dive deep into the scientific evidence, share insight into my clinical experience with fasting, and finally lay out a wide number of fasting strategies for you to implement into your life.

While not every person will be able to utilize the same fasting strategy, everyone can implement some form of fasting into their life with great benefit.

History of Fasting

Fasting is the oldest, most inexpensive, and arguably most powerful healing strategy known to man.

Fasting likely first occurred as an adaptation to hunter gatherer lifestyles lived by our ancestors. Let's face it, when you have to chase down an animal or rummage through the woods for some berries to feed a tribe – you might go a few days at a time without food.

Our ancient ancestors did not have easy access to food. As hunters and gatherers, they would often go days and in some cases weeks with very little food. As we developed agricultural practices, there were many dry seasons and poor harvests which meant less than adequate food for the civilization.

Our ancestors didn't have refrigeration or modern ways of storing food so when they did kill an animal or had a successful harvest they would feast for days until the food was gone.

This sort of feast-famine cycling was imprinted into our DNA. Our bodies are built for survival and are remarkably good at going long periods of time without food. If we had to depend upon eating every day (much less multiple meals each day), humanity would not have survived our early years.

It appears though, that once humans adapted and solved the problem of food scarcity through animal domestication and agricultural practices – some humans still chose to partake in fasting practices for perceived health benefits.

Ancient warriors and hunters even realized that they had more drive and had greater strength and endurance when they went to war or on the hunt in a semi fasted state. They had greater "hunger" and improved mental focus which is one of the key fasting benefits you will learn about in this book.

It just so happens that modern science has uncovered powerful benefits of fasting that reaffirm what some of our ancestors were feeling. Science is showing us that fasting restores strength to the immune system, restores the vitality of just about every cell in the human body, and heightens your mental state. It makes you healthier, extends lifespan, and its free.

The Ancient Greeks

As civilizations developed, we were able to advance our agricultural practices and learned more sophisticated ways to store food. This led to less famine and greater food abundance. Some cultures had access to food all year round. However, many of the philosophers, doctors and religious leaders still advocated for fasting as a way to improve our physical, mental and spiritual health.

The Greek historian Herodotus (484–425 BC), believed the Egyptians to be much healthier than the Greeks due to their regular fasting practices. He was quoted as saying that "the Egyptians are the healthiest of men, since each month for 3 days they conduct purification by vomiting and enemas, believing that a person receives all illness through food."

Hippocrates, the Father of Modern Medicine, once said "The addition of food should be much rarer, since it is often useful to completely take it away while the patient can withstand it, until the force of the disease reaches its maturity. The man carries within him a doctor; you just have to help him do his work. If the body is not cleared, then the more you feed it, the more it will be harmed. When a patient is fed too richly, the disease is fed as well. Remember – any excess is against nature."

The Greek philosopher Plato said, "I fast for greater mental and physical efficiency." He was saying that he felt as though fasting helped him be more efficient with both his mental and physical energy. The research shows that Plato was correct in that fasting improves both our metabolic flexibility and energy efficiency.

Fasting in Spiritual and Biblical Context

Fasting is revered in almost every major religion. It is used as a way to transcend the limits of the physical body and grow spiritually as well as mourn the loss of loved ones. In addition, many use the practice of fasting to seek wisdom and clarity on specific matters.

In Judaism, followers fast without food or water on Yom Kippur (The Day of Atonement). This practice is thought to help the individual atone for their sins and sacrifice the needs of their flesh to please God. This is typically a 24-hour period from sundown on the first day until sundown on the second day.

Muslims fast each year during Ramadan, the ninth month of the Islamic calendar. During this time, they fast from food and water during daylight hours. It is usually 12 hours on average, however, in some regions, it may be up to 22 hours per day.

In Christianity, fasting happens during Lent and Advent, where some members will even fast from food for up to 40 days as a way of participating in Christ's sacrificial life and death on the cross.

In Mormonism, many members will fast on one Sunday of each month. In Buddhism, people use fasting to aid meditation, and in Jainism, to reach transcendence. Jewish, Mormon, and Islamic fasts are dry fasts since they prohibit water along with food as well.

In biblical days, fasting was a normal part of a spiritual life. Jesus fasted for 40 days before beginning his ministry. Many of the prophets discussed fasting and Jesus, when talking to his disciples and followers said "When you fast..." This was discussed using the terminology as though fasting was a normal way of life for the Hebrew people.

Here are some of the many references out of the bible for fasting.

"Moses neither ate bread, nor drank water for forty days and forty nights." (Exodus 34:28)

"Esther calls all Jewish people everywhere to neither eat nor drink for three days, night or day." (Esther 4:16)

"The king of Nineveh repents and declares that people and animals do a dry fast." (Jonah 3:7-8)

"Is not this the kind of fasting I have chosen: to loose the chains of injustice and untie the cords of the yoke, to set the oppressed free and break every yoke?" (Isaiah 58:6)

"So we fasted and petitioned our God about this, and he answered our prayer." (Ezra 8:23)

"So after they had fasted and prayed, they placed their hands on them and sent them off." (Acts 13:3)

"When you fast, do not look somber as the hypocrites do, for they disfigure their faces to show others they are fasting. Truly I tell you, they have received their reward in full." (Matthew 6:16)

It’s Time to Break the Societal Programming

Fasting was essential for our survival as a species, it has been built into our DNA since we’ve existed on this planet, and science has confirmed numerous health benefits.

The only challenge we have left to address as a society is the societal programming that tells us we need to have 3 meals a day and snacks in between. We have to liberate ourselves from the idea that we are going to starve if we skip a meal.

Metabolic diseases are one of the biggest controllable threats to humankind. They kill more people than anything else, they are expensive to treat in the medical system, they predispose you to infectious disease, YET THEY ARE COMPLETELY CONTROLLABLE THROUGH LIFESTYLE... FOR FREE!

This should be exciting and liberating news!

Now it’s time to break some misconceptions and lay down the science.

Fasting is NOT Starvation

Right out of the gate, there is a major misconception I want to break... fasting and starvation are not the same thing. In fact, there are three important distinctions to be made before we get started: Caloric Restriction Vs. Fasting Vs. Starvation.

Caloric Restriction is simply consuming less calories than your body requires on a daily basis. This has been the predominant basis for weight loss programs for many years. Caloric restriction has been shown to improve many aspects of health and improve lifespan in almost all species.

Fasting refers to a period of time in which zero calories are consumed. For example, most everyone is fasting while they sleep! There are many different types of fasting but one that is very popular is intermittent fasting, also referred to as time-restricted eating. Most types of fasting will influence the body to shift closer to a state of ketosis while caloric restriction doesn’t necessarily do this.

This is where someone skips breakfast and reserves all of their eating to later in the day – for example from 2pm-6pm. This is a 4-hour eating window which means the individual fasts for the remaining 20 hours outside of that window.

An important distinction to make with fasting is that, depending on your goals, you can still consume enough calories in this window to put on weight. Fasting will still require a caloric deficit to elicit weight loss.

Starvation is when the body takes in very few calories for an extended period and the body is not able to maintain normal metabolic processes.

Signs of starvation include weakness, muscle wasting, apathy, and loss of menstruation in females. In stark contrast to fasting, people generally feel energized and preserve muscle tissue quit well in the presence of adequate calories and nutrients.

Past vs Current Uses for Fasting

This might start to sound repetitive, but it is important to understand. If we think back to our ancestors and how they lived their lives, fasting was likely a part of everyday operations. In the time of hunter gatherers, before we invented modern day agriculture, it was normal to eat when food was available and fast when it was not.

In fact, it was likely fasting that kept us alive in times when food was scarce. Not only did the human body adapt to be able to survive in a fasted state, but it actually seems like most humans see profound health benefits from going into a fasted state periodically.

We'll cover many reasons for why this might be the case throughout the book. The main point I want to get across right now is that you should not feel like you are doing anything out of the ordinary if you choose to adopt a fasting routine.

So, when you get crazy looks and questions of concern from friends or family about your new fasting routine, you can tell them it's completely natural! You are NOT starving yourself; you are harnessing one of the most powerful healing tools humans have developed.

Just like any tool, fasting can be abused. Take proper planning steps to ensure you are receiving adequate nutrition outside of the fasting window.

In addition to fasting due to food scarcity, we previously discussed how there are a number of records of people intentionally fasting for a wide range of benefits.

Before we understood much of the scientific basis of fasting, it was understood that fasting could be used as a tool to gain heightened mental clarity and even be used as a tool to achieve higher levels of spiritual enlightenment.

This is likely due to shifting into a state of ketosis that provides the brain with a stable supply of ketones that calm the mind and provide a state of calm focus that is difficult to obtain otherwise. During these periods of heightened mental clarity, people claimed to be able to access higher levels of consciousness and obtain profound insights.

While people still partake in fasting for religious and spiritual reasons, it is also common for people to adopt fasting as a means of improving chronic disease, supporting mental health and performance, and even to assist in addiction resolution.

Now that you are aware of the history of fasting, let's dive into what some of the potential benefits are. We will also go over how to incorporate both intermittent fasting, partial fasting and extended fasting strategies. Finally, you will learn how to trouble shoot the most common challenges people have when they begin a fasting lifestyle.

Chapter 1: The Benefits of Fasting

A vast proportion of modern-day disease is related to metabolic dysfunction. Metabolic diseases include diabetes, obesity, heart disease, and cancer. The cost of global metabolic disease is estimated to be in the trillions of dollars (1).

What you may not know is that one of the first fundamental failures that occurs in the body leading to metabolic disease is insulin resistance. This is when cells stop responding to the stimulus of insulin and sugar is not able to get into the cells. When sugar is not being used by cells, it is much more likely to get converted into fat.

When sugar does not make it into cells, the brain up regulates appetite because it thinks the body is not receiving adequate nutrition. This leads to a chronic cycle of overeating and appetite dysregulation. Luckily, fasting may be one of the most efficient ways of restoring insulin sensitivity and burning fat.

Healing the Metabolism and Burning Fat

When you begin fasting, your body goes through distinct metabolic shifts. First, you burn off glycogen stores from the liver. Once glycogen has been utilized, the body will begin mobilizing fat, converting it into ketones, then using those ketones as a source of energy.

The more often you fast, the more quickly the body will shift into fat burning in the absence of sugar. When you have the ability to quickly switch between sugar and fat stores as an energy source, you are considered metabolically flexible and have become very energy efficient.

Metabolic Flexibility: The ability to change our metabolism to meet the demands of our environment.

Energy Efficiency: Using our energy in the most efficient matter possible to regulate all the needs of the body.

Having both metabolic flexibility and energy efficiency programed within your biology allows you to stay healthy effortlessly and get more done in your daily life.

The traditional weight loss strategy is to consume several meals a day while restricting calories to keep the metabolism up. It turns out that this approach may actually have the opposite effect. Chronically restricting calories in the absence of fasting tends to actually reduce metabolic rate (2, 3).

Fasting promotes fat burning through a massive surge in growth hormone (4). Additionally, fasting promotes insulin sensitivity and therefore a more efficient utilization of energy by the body (5).

Restoring Insulin Sensitivity

When you eat something with carbohydrates in it, the carbohydrates are converted into glucose and shuttled into cells with the help of insulin. A rise in insulin levels signals the body to *burn sugar* and *store fat.*

Chronic elevation in insulin due to eating too often or overconsumption of carbohydrates can lead to cells that no longer respond to insulin – leading you to have low energy, always being hungry, and chronic inflammation. Fasting is able to restore insulin's reaction with your cells, so appetite is controlled and less fat storage occurs (6).

Another interesting benefit to note is that insulin delivers certain nutrients to your cells – such as magnesium. Magnesium is required for over 300 functions in the human body and without adequate amounts there can be several issues.

Fasting helps to reestablish cellular nutrient levels by improving transportation through insulin receptors. Having optimal insulin sensitivity is critical to ensure many of the nutrients you are eating actually make it into your cells!

Signs of Insulin Resistance

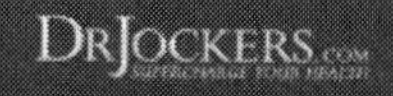

- Tend to Be Overweight
- Trouble Losing Weight
- Large Appetite
- Craving Sweets After Meals
- Eating Sweets Dosn't Relieve Cravings
- Feeling More Tired After Meals
- Frequent Thirst and Urge to Urinate
- Hormone Problems - PCOS
- Females - Estrogen or Testosterone Dominance
- Males - Low Testosterone
- Acne, Skin Tags and Skin Pigmentation Changes
- High Blood Pressure and High Triglycerides

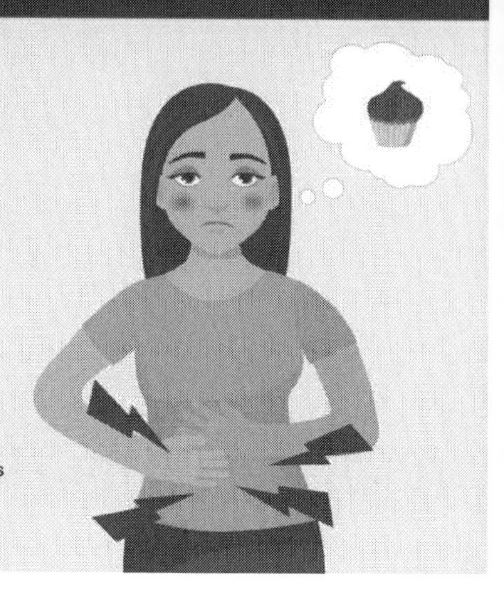

Ultimate Anti-Inflammatory

Chronic inflammation is a hallmark of just about every chronic disease known to man. Inflammation isn't entirely bad though; its role is to direct the immune system towards places in the body that need healing or immune support so that the body can resolve issues.

Self-inducing chronic inflammation through lifestyle is a major problem, however. When we are constantly eating inflammatory foods or overeating, we are only increasing inflammation and creating a greater burden on our metabolisms.

One study on Ramadan fasting observed a reduction in pro-inflammatory cytokine concentrations during fasting periods (7). Elevations in pro-inflammatory cytokines are indicated in metabolic syndrome, cancer, arthritis, chronic pain, and heart disease (8, 9, 10).

Another study showed that fasting for 16 hours a day produced a significant reduction in neuro inflammasomes over a 4-month period (11). These are genetic receptors that are heavily involved in eliciting inflammation within the brain. This study was performed on ischemic stroke patients who had high levels of neuro-inflammation.

Perhaps, by down regulating inflammatory processes in the brain, we are able to limit our chances of succumbing to neuro-degenerative diseases such as dementia, Alzheimer's, and Parkinson's.

Cellular Autophagy

In the 1960's, researchers noticed that cells were able to destroy themselves and recycle parts to make new cells. This process, named autophagy, is a critical role of the immune system. Through autophagy, the body is able identify and destroy weak and malfunctioning cells yet conserve parts of these cells that were still good to rebuild new cells.

Autophagy is essentially how our body stays young. This is how we build new organ tissue and heal from disease.

In fact, disruption of autophagy is considered a major contributor to neurodegenerative disease (12).

One key aspect of autophagy that is important to mention is mitophagy. Mitophagy is the break down and recycling of mitochondria specifically. This is absolutely necessary considering your mitochondria produce all of the energy your body requires for sustaining life.

Without autophagy, we would not live very long as humans. Fasting is one of the best ways to assist the body in performing autophagy and prevent several diseases (13).

Stem Cells

Right now, there is a massive trend going on in stem cell research and treatment for just about every disease known to man. This makes perfect sense because stem cells can be guided and directed to heal damaged areas of the body. This means that a metabolically healthy body with plenty of stem cells should have no problem healing damaged tissues.

A stem cell is essentially a cell that has not been assigned to a given role in the body yet. Before a cell becomes a liver, muscle, or brain cell – it is first a stem cell. Your body constantly produces stem cells in order to direct them to areas that are in need of regeneration.

The importance of stem cells is similar to the importance of the mitochondria that I just briefly discussed in the autophagy section. In fact, autophagy and stem cell direction by the body are complimentary processes vital for staying healthy.

It makes sense then that fasting not only improves autophagy, but also up-regulates stem cell activity. The level of stem cell activity seems to be dependent on the length of the fast where longer fasting periods tend to stimulate higher levels of stem cells.

That being said, it also seems that this effect is dependent on the life cycle of cells in a given tissue. For example, cells in the intestine regenerate every 3-5 days whereas cells in the liver may take 6 months to a year or longer to regenerate. Perhaps many of the benefits of fasting come from the acceleration of stem cell production and tissue renewal cycles.

Studies in mice and humans have shown that prolonged fasting (48-120 hours) reduces Insulin like growth factor -1 (IGF-1) and Protein Kinase A (PKA)(14). These are pro-growth signaling molecules that are not inherently bad, but can promote cancer and shorten lifespan if they are not kept under control. Instead fasting activates alternative pathways that help your cells protect themselves from toxins and stress.

Another significant application of prolonged fasting is the reduction in certain chemotherapy side effects. One study found that prolonged fasting combined with chemotherapy can increase hematopoietic stem cells, which may help prevent the dangerous immunosuppression that often comes along with chemotherapy treatment (15).

While stem cell injections may seem enticing, just remember that your body has the ability to up-regulate its own stem cells – FOR FREE!

Youthful Hormones

One of the main hormones thought to keep the body young is human growth hormone (also known as HGH). HGH signals the body to repair damaged cells, stimulate fat burning, support lean muscle growth, keep the bones strong, and keep the immune system in balance.

In addition to everything above, having balanced HGH levels also helps to improve joint and skin health by improving collagen synthesis.

Fasting is likely one of the most impactful strategies for increasing HGH. This conclusion is based on a study done at the Intermountain Medical Center which studied men and women as they implemented 24-hour fasting periods. What they found was that at the end of the 24-hour period, men had an increase of 2000% while women had an increase of 1300% in HGH (16).

This increase in HGH is unseen in any other non-drug-based interventional strategies.

Reduce Chronic Disease Risk

The top killers of humans worldwide are chronic diseases that are highly attributed to lifestyle choices. It is easy to draw this conclusion because they are mostly diseases of the metabolism. Metabolic disorders include type 2 diabetes, obesity, heart disease, stroke, and high blood pressure.

It is estimated that a quarter of the world's population has metabolic syndrome (17).

Seriously think about that for a second... A quarter of the world's population—nearly 2 billion people (at the time of this writing)—may be dealing with metabolic syndrome. The peripheral effects of metabolic syndrome on our economic system are estimated to be in the TRILLIONS.

Metabolic conditions may be the single biggest stressor on our healthcare systems. Having metabolic syndrome sets you at a higher predisposition of dying from any cause. When it comes down to it, metabolic syndrome is a disease of energy mismanagement. When your body does not manage energy well you don't bounce back from health ailments as easily.

When you are metabolically damaged, it may even take you longer to spring back from things like injuries and infections.

One of the simplest, yet free, interventions for getting our chronic disease epidemic under control may be promoting a fasting lifestyle. Preliminary studies show that fasting improves insulin sensitivity, body fat levels, blood pressure, control over stress (measured by heart rate variability), inflammation levels, and protective effects against brain and heart damage (18).

Improved Relationship with Food

Mindless eating, hourly snacking, and sugar cravings are common. Next time you're at work or even around your own family, observe eating patterns. You'll start to notice that between meals, snack, and beverages; some people have virtually zero breaks from calories all day long. Fasting is the fastest to realize how palliative our food dependence is.

The most difficult part about adopting a fasting lifestyle is simply breaking mental and emotional dependencies that we develop by abusing food on a regular basis.

Many people feel deprived when they first begin fasting. In some cases, you may be able to consider this sensation a withdrawal from food. This is a sign that food has become a drug used to either stimulate certain feelings or avoid feeling others.

Fasting and getting through these temporary feelings is one of the quickest ways to reset your psychological dependence and become more mindful of your relationship with food.

Mental Health and Focus

In addition to the emotional and psychological benefits of improving your relationship with food, there are physiological explanations for the mental benefits of fasting.

For example, when you fast for long enough your body will deplete its glycogen stores and begin to burn body fat for energy. This is known as ketosis. Once entering this state, most people say they feel energetic, yet calm and focused. Additionally, they say they can so several hours without feeling hungry or even thinking about food.

This is because your body takes stored fat and converts it into ketones. Ketones provide a more stable and long-lasting energy compared to sugar. From a subjective standpoint I often hear the following about burning sugar vs. burning ketones as a primary energy source:

"Before I tried fasting, I did what I thought was right for my metabolism—3–6 balanced meals a day with carbs, protein, and fat. I often found myself obsessed over my next meal with very distinct raises and drops in my energy levels... Everyone around me knew when I hadn't eaten in a while because I would just get cranky. Since I've been fasting it's like I can go all day and not even think about food or experience a dip in energy! I almost can't believe that I was told to do the opposite all this time. My energy levels have stabilized and I'm mentally clear finally."

This experience is so common. I mean, who hasn't read the food pyramid guidelines? I remember these being drilled into my head as an elementary school student and thinking that pizza with vegetables was a "balanced meal." Ridiculous!

Luckily, we know better now. It is easy for me to feel that I am most mentally clear and do my best work when I am fasted. I also feel more resilient to stress and generally at peace.

Intermittent fasting is likely one of the best ways to maintain daily cognitive sharpness while prolonged fasting shows promise for more clinical mental health issues. A 2013 review published in Psychiatry Research showed that a prolonged fast over 7 days was able to improve mood, alertness, and subjective sense of tranquility in clinical depression (19).

Improved Energy

Once you are adapted to fasting, you will likely experience more energy and level energy throughout the day. This mostly due to shifting the body into a state of ketosis which:

1. Provides an efficient energy source, Ketones
2. Promotes the recycling of damaged mitochondria, Mitophagy
3. Increases the production of new mitochondria, Mitochondrial Biogenesis

Once you have become efficient at burning ketones for energy, you will generate more ATP and
less oxidative stress at a cellular level. This means more energy and less inflammation. I often relate the difference in sugar metabolism vs ketone metabolism to standard vs premium fuel in a car. They both produce energy, but one gets better miles per gallon and produces less toxic waste!

In addition to having cleaner burning fuel, we have the generation of more efficient and resilient mitochondria to burn that fuel.

Another aspect of fasting that may provide energy benefit is a notable increase in norepinephrine. Norepinephrine is a stimulating hormone with the function of increasing mental alertness and energy availability in the cells.

Overall, the mechanisms above synergize with one another to provide a heightened state of wellbeing.

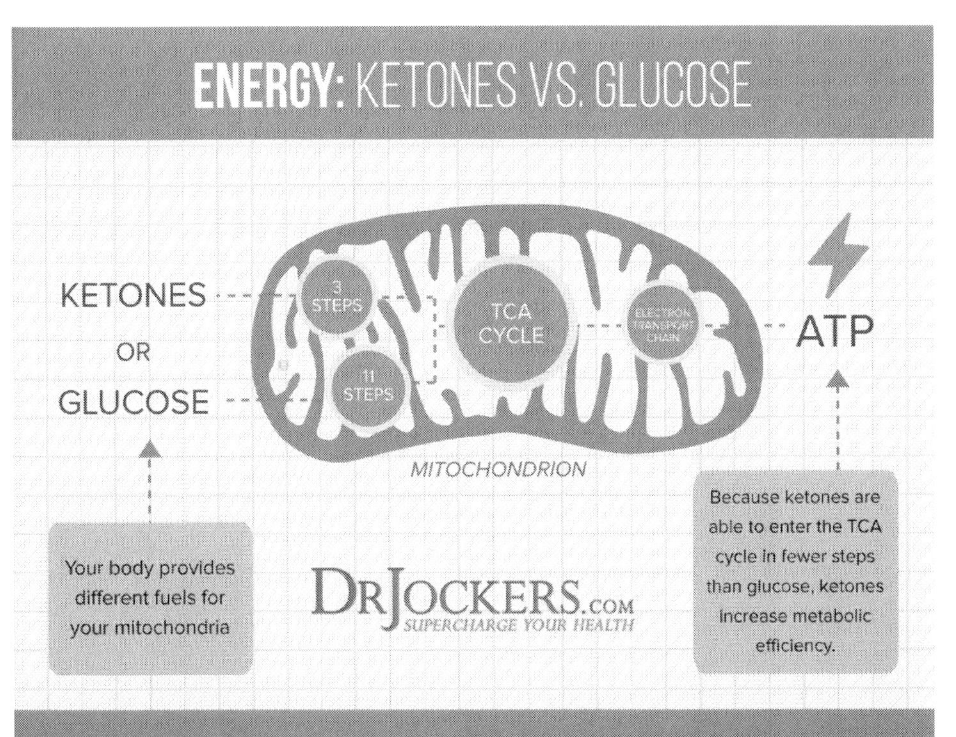

Healing the Digestive System

Digestion is an energy-demanding process in the body. If you think about it, most modern-day humans never give their digestive tract a break. Between the several hours it takes to digest food and fully eliminate waste, some people may go years without giving their gut more than a couple hours to regenerate itself.

In addition to never giving digestion a break, most humans frequently consume things that are inflammatory to the gut including: grains, alcohol, chemically treated tap water, non-organic produce, and certain medications.

Fasting allows the body to delegate this energy elsewhere while also allowing the intestinal walls some time to rebuild.

Digestive issues are often at the root of chronic diseases like autoimmunity, skin disorders, and unwanted mental conditions such as anxiety and depression.

In fact, in my health coaching and Functional Medicine practice, it very rare to find someone that is not dealing with concerning digestive symptoms. I would recommend not taking digestive symptoms lightly, they are often a preliminary sign that something is off within your body.

Luckily, the intestinal lining repairs itself rather quickly. In fact, a 2018 study showed that a 24 hour fast stimulated an increase in intestinal stem cell production (20). In my clinical experience, fasting is one of the most powerful strategies for healing the body whether there are digestive issues present or not.

Heightened Intuition, Spiritual Guidance, Decision Making

As I have mentioned already, fasting has been used throughout history to heighten mental attentiveness. It has been used by every major religion and spiritual practice in order to increase connection with divine sources of guidance. Even major innovators responsible for great accomplishments have been known to fast leading up to major mental breakthroughs.

Many people report being able to connect deeper with their inner voice of truth and feel grounded in their daily decision making knowing that they are making decisions in a clear mind free from distraction.

It may come down to the fact that without the constant draw to external stimuli, we are able to pinpoint the decisions and behaviors that are really important in life. We are able to identify and shed behaviors that we partake in as distractions from other problems in our lives, allowing us to rebuild a clear vision on what we really want in life.

No matter your beliefs, progress in life requires a vision. Developing a vision requires the ability to focus on what is important. Fasting provides stable energy and a clear mind to help you develop your vision. It also helps you identify destructive behaviors that are holding you back from seeing that vision. Fasting is the epitome of self-development when implemented in this way.

The Global Metabolic Pandemic (and Why Everyone Should Consider Adopting a Fasting Lifestyle)

Hopefully by now you understand just how powerful to have some kind of fasting practice in your life. Even a small daily fast can provide health and performance benefits.

Before we get into the application and implementation of fasting strategies, I want to make one more major point... Humans are suffering. I know it's straight to the point and not fun to think about but it's true.

We are living longer than ever yet we all have loved ones who have gone through the downward spiral of chronic disease, summing it all up to old age. We need powerful healing strategies that are easy to implement and efficient.

I believe fasting is one of the best tools we've had and we need to make sure people know about it. Here's why.

Diseases of the metabolism are the number one cause of death in the world. According to the Centers for Disease Control and Prevention National Center for Health Statistics, the leading causes of death in the US are:

1. Heart Disease
2. Cancer
3. Unintentional Injuries and Accidents
4. Chronic Lower Respiratory Diseases
5. Alzheimer's Disease
6. Diabetes
7. Flu and Pneumonia
8. Kidney Disease
9. Suicide

These statistics aren't just true for the US. Statistics show that we are starting to see metabolic disease trending upward worldwide. As we develop new technology and provide under-developed countries with more resources, we start to see the same diseases. Diseases of excess.

Based on the benefits of having a balanced metabolism that I have laid out so far, it is hard to imagine that adopting a fasting-focused lifestyle couldn't dramatically alter each and every one of these statistics in a beneficial way.

In addition to being highly impactful against a wide array of ailments, fasting is free and relatively easy to implement. You simply stop eating for a time frame you are comfortable with and repeat as necessary.

Later in this book we will cover a number of fasting strategies that can be suited to a variety of needs including:

- Intermittent or Daily Fasting
- Weekly Fasting Cycles
- Partial Fasting and Fasting Mimicking Diets
- Prolonged Fasts (48 Hours or more)
- Applications for Different Diseases
- ...and how to troubleshoot the process of becoming metabolically flexible

Before we dive in, I want to emphasize that it is still incredibly important to focus on the quality of foods you are eating when you are not fasting. This is not a miracle fix for a bad diet. Fasting and good nutrition go hand-in-hand and I've personally witnessed massive changes in peoples' lives by combining the two.

I have hundreds of comprehensive nutrition articles available on my website Drjockers.com and provide health coaching services including functional lab work evaluation for anyone looking to dive deeper into what optimal nutrition and lifestyle could mean for you.

I also wrote an entire book on optimizing the metabolism through nutrition titled **Keto Metabolic Breakthrough** which dives into using ketogenic diet principles to limit inflammation, promote healing, and restore your metabolism.

For this book, we are taking a deep dive into fasting, its benefits, and different fasting strategies that can be implemented to suit your goals and needs.

By the end of this book you will be equipped with the knowledge to design the exact fasting protocol for your goals.

Chapter 2: The Science Behind Fasting

Now you understand just how far back fasting goes in our ancestry. Not only is fasting built into our DNA, but it is likely one of the most powerful mechanisms for healing in the human body. When your body realizes there is no external food coming in for a while, it shifts into a more energy efficient metabolism and deep healing occurs.

So far, we have laid down a condensed but significant history of fasting. We've also covered a wide range of powerful benefits that come along with partaking in abstinence from food.

Now I want to take a dive into some of the more technical science.

When it comes to fasting, there are 5 major mechanisms that seem to stand out that explain many of the benefits:

1. Insulin Sensitivity – Allowing Better Regulation of Blood Sugar and Cell Energy Balance
2. Stimulating Ketosis – Shifting the Body Away from Sugar Metabolism to Fat Metabolism
3. Human Growth Hormone (HGH) – Promoting Cell Regeneration and Growth
4. AMPk – Promoting Fat Burning, Cell Recycling through Autophagy, and Stimulating the Growth of New Mitochondria
5. Stem Cells – Cells that Can Be Directed to Damaged Tissues to Promote Regeneration

Now let's define each of these mechanisms and learn a bit more about how fasting can affect them.

Fasting Mechanism: Insulin Sensitivity

Insulin is a hormone that allows glucose in the blood to enter cells. Insulin sensitivity is a measure of the relative amount of insulin needed for this process to occur. In other words, how sensitive your cells are to insulin signals.

When relatively little amounts of insulin are needed to allow glucose into cells, this would be considered a high amount of insulin sensitivity (this is a good thing). This is when you eat a meal, your blood sugar rises temporarily, and insulin is able to efficiently place sugar into your cells – returning your blood sugar back to normal without any significant changes in energy.

When relatively high amounts of insulin are needed to allow glucose into cells, this would be considered a low amount of insulin sensitivity (also known as insulin resistance). Instead of your meals being efficiently processed into glucose and shuttled into your cells, glucose remains in the blood and your cells are left in an energy deprived state. Next, I will cover some of the main causes and symptoms of insulin problems in addition to why you should always ensure your insulin levels stay balanced.

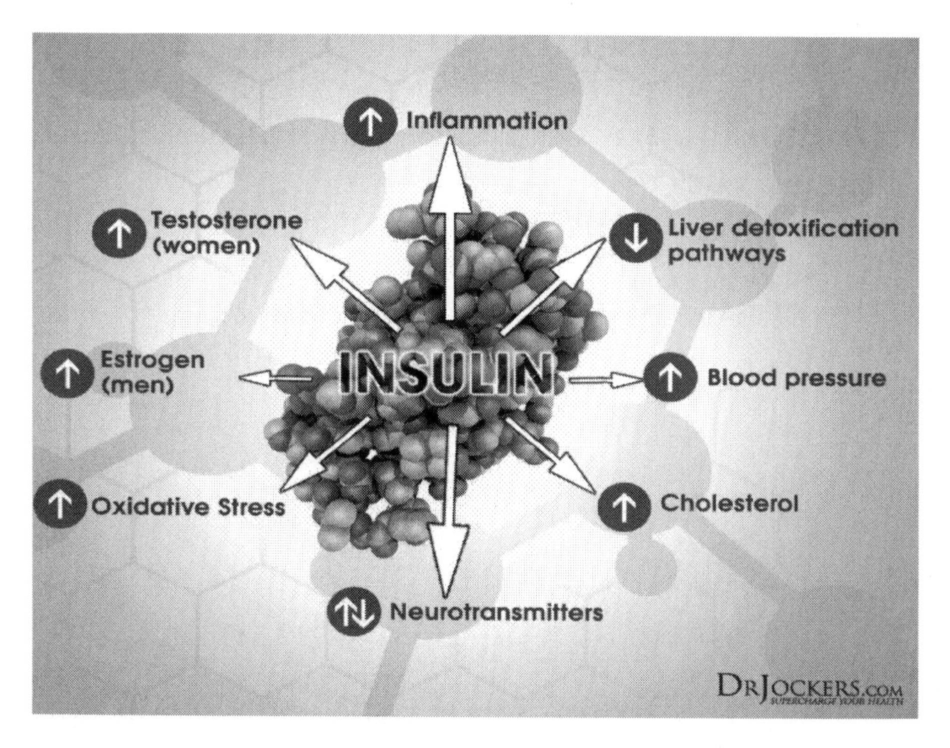

Insulin Resistance

As stated above, insulin resistance is when cells do not respond adequately to insulin. The result of this is that glucose in the blood is not able to enter cells. When excess glucose is left circulating in the blood, the body tries to compensate by converting it into fat that can be stored for later use.

This is why you often find that those with insulin resistance also find themselves with abdominal obesity, fatty liver disease, elevated triglycerides, or other fat deposits.

The development of insulin resistance is progressive, eventually leading to prediabetes and type II diabetes if left uncontrolled (1).

Additionally, the development of insulin resistance often also raises your risk of the following:

- High Blood Pressure
- Heart Disease
- Stroke
- Liver Failure
- Dementia
- Certain Cancers
- Metabolic Syndrome
- Mood Disorders
- ...and likely A LOT more

Ultimately, the repercussions of having a malfunctioning metabolism are incredibly wide-ranging and impact every major mechanism of accelerated aging (2). Perhaps this is why fasting has been shown to extend lifespan!

Symptoms of Insulin Resistance

As I just reviewed, insulin resistance can really cause a lot of problems in the body. In addition to the diseases listed above, there are several symptoms that signify insulin resistance such as:

- Abdominal Obesity
- Insatiable Appetite
- Feeling Tired After Meals
- Weight Loss Resistance
- Craving Sweets After Meals
- Frequent Thirst and Urination

- Estrogen or Testosterone Dominance (Females)
- Low Testosterone (Males)
- Chronic Skin Issues
- High Triglycerides
- High Blood Pressure
- Anxiety Upon Missing a Meal

How to Measure if You Are Insulin Resistant

There are several ways to test yourself for insulin resistance and get an idea of your blood sugar balance. If you have several of the symptoms listed above, you may want to consider some of the tests below. Also keep in mind that it will not always be obvious if someone is in the process of becoming insulin resistant.

It is possible to go years not knowing you are insulin resistant! Considering blood sugar balance (glycemic control) has been identified as one of the primary determining factors in health and longevity, you may consider having these markers tested on a fairly regular basis.

Hemoglobin A1C (HbA1C)

The hemoglobin A1C (HbA1C) test indicates what your blood glucose levels have been over the last 90 days. Hemoglobin (Hb) is a component of your red blood cells that undergoes a reaction called glycation when it interacts with excess glucose in the blood. When this reaction occurs, it becomes HbA1C. The higher your blood sugar, the more Hb will react with it to become HbA1C (3, 4, 5)

Since red blood cells have a lifecycle of about 90 days, measuring your HbA1C levels is a great way to get a snapshot of your glycemic control.

When this test is used to classify insulin resistance levels, a percentage is created between Hb molecules that have been glycated by sugar and Hb molecules that are normal. The following are generally accepted clinical ranges for HbA1C:

- **Normal HbA1C:** Healthy levels of HbA1C are under 5.6 percent. Most functional and holistic medicine doctors prefer to see them under 5.2 percent in order to stay on the safe and healthy side.
- **Prediabetes:** Between 5.7 and 6.5 percent is when prediabetes is diagnosed.
- **Diabetes:** Over 6.5 percent is when diabetes is diagnosed.

Fasting Plasma Glucose Test (FPG)

As the name of the test implies, the Fasting Plasma Glucose test measures blood sugar levels while you are in a fasted state. When performed clinically, most doctors advise skipping breakfast and having the test performed mid-morning to allow for a minimum of 8 hours since the previous meal.

If blood sugar remains elevated 8 or more hours after your last meal, this is a sign of insulin resistance.

The following are generally accepted clinical ranges for Fasting Plasma Glucose:

- **Normal FPG:** Under 100 mg/dl is considered normal, though functional and holistic medicine doctors prefer to see this number under 90 mg/dl.
- **Prediabetes:** Between 100 and 126 mg/dl, is considered prediabetic.
- **Diabetes:** Over 126 mg/dl, diabetes is diagnosed.

Oral Glucose Tolerance Test (OGTT)

The OGTT measures how your body responds to a dose of sugar. Starting in a fasted state, you are instructed to consume a 75-gram dose of glucose within a 5-minute window. Following the consumption of glucose, a doctor will take a series of blood glucose measurements immediately after, two hours following, and sometimes several hours later.

If your blood sugar remains elevated hours after consuming glucose, this us a great indicator that you are insulin resistant.

The advantage of this type of test is that it can identify certain problems earlier than a fasting glucose test can.

The following are generally accepted clinical ranges for an Oral Glucose Tolerance Test at the 2-hour mark:

- **Normal OGTT:** Normal levels are considered to be under 140 mg/dl, though functional and holistic medicine doctors prefer to see numbers under 120 mg/dl.
- **Prediabetes:** A range from 140 to 200 mg/dl is considered prediabetic.
- **Diabetes:** Anything over 200 mg/dl is considered diabetes.

Continuous Blood Glucose Monitor

Another great way to measure your blood sugar levels is to wear a continuous blood glucose monitor. This is a minimally invasive monitor, often attached to the back of the arm, that monitors your blood sugar levels throughout the day.

The advantage of this technology is that you can get a much better idea of what your blood sugar looks like throughout the day and you can keep track of trends over several weeks. This way, you can track in real-time if interventional strategies, such as fasting or exercise, are helping you.

Two popular options for this are the Freestyle Libre device as well as the Dexcom C6.

The Negative Feedback Loop of Energy Balance and Why Fasting is the Single Best Solution for Insulin Resistance

Now I want to cover why fasting is likely one of the best tools for restoring insulin sensitivity.

Dr. Jason Fung, one of the leading researchers on the subject of fasting and Type II Diabetes, summarizes the process of insulin resistance very well.

He states that energy production in a cell is similar to filling your car up with gasoline. You have a tank that holds a set amount of fuel to create energy. The gas pump has a built-in mechanism that shuts off the flow of gas when the tank is full. Once the tank is full, the only way to pump more gas into the tank is if you drive around for a while to burn it up.

Similar to how a gas tank works in a car, your cells can only metabolize so much glucose at a given time. When too much glucose builds up within a cell, it effectively begins to overflow and become increasingly concentrated within the blood. Your pancreas then raises insulin levels to try and maintain blood sugar balance, but the already saturated cells cannot take in any more glucose. Your cells then counteract glucose flow into cells by shutting down insulin receptor activity, hence insulin resistance.

So then, if we retrace the cascade of insulin resistance, we can see the first step of the process is an **abundance of glucose**. That being said, an abundance of fats or proteins can also lead to this energy excess and promote the buildup of glucose as well.

The first step in addressing this cascade is drastically reducing glucose supply to allow for the metabolism of what is currently available.

The most efficient way to do this is fasting.

Here's What the Science Says...

In rodent models, time-restricted feeding (TRF) has been shown to prevent and even cure Type II diabetes.

One study published in the International Journal of Molecular Medicine demonstrated just that (6). Rats were given a hyper-caloric diet until they developed insulin resistance and diabetes. Basically, they were allowed to eat whenever they wanted and however much they wanted. The researchers then took one group of the diabetic rats and placed them on a TRF schedule that only made food available to the rats for 8 hours out of the day.

What they saw in this study was a reversal of insulin resistance and Diabetes as long as the TRF schedule was maintained.

Another rodent study in 2012 reconstructing similar conditions showed that an 8-hour feeding window was able to reverse insulin resistance, obesity, and systemic inflammation (7). **What was really interesting about this study is that they did not control for caloric intake. This suggests that independent of how many calories you consume, simply fasting periodically can have favorable effects on your insulin requirements and metabolic health.**

In rodent models, daily fasting has also demonstrated:

- The ability to protect the heart tissue from myocardial infarction damage (8)
- Improved survival and heart function following a major heart attack (9)
- Protection against age-related fibrosis and inflammation (10)
- Reduction in blood pressure (11)
- Improvement in cholesterol and triglycerides (12, 13, 14)
- Protection against stroke (15)

All of the above outcomes point to beneficial changes in insulin sensitivity and the metabolic processes of the body.

In addition to the benefits above, there have been several studies that have demonstrated that prolonged fasting of 2 or more days was as effective as chemotherapy for delaying cancer development. Additionally, fasting was able to protect healthy cells from the damaging effects of chemotherapy while also aiding in the destruction of cancer cells (16).

As you can see, there is a robust base of evidence supporting the benefits of fasting in animal studies. In fact, fasting has been shown to increase lifespan in just about every species studied!

So, do these benefits apply to humans as well?

A recent review of fasting research in humans determined that on average an Alternate-Day fasting routine achieved (17):

- Reduction in Body Fat
- Weight Loss
- Reduction in Triglyceride Levels
- And Improved Insulin Sensitivity (18)

Another large review of available evidence in 2017 concluded that intermittent fasting is protective against metabolic disease, diabetes, and heart disease (19).

While the majority of fasting studies have been performed on animals, it seems apparent that fasting is both safe for humans and great tool for restoring health.

In my clinical experience I have observed hundreds of people change their lives using daily or prolonged fasting strategies. From the perspective of insulin sensitivity, I offer direct-to-consumer lab testing that tracks several indicators of metabolic health that might not always be tested by a medical doctor.

On my website drjockers.com you can check out my Lab Testing page where I offer an in-depth blood work analysis that includes markers of metabolic health mentioned above. Alternatively, you can request the markers above from your doctor next time you have routine lab work done!

I have observed first-hand that fasting is able to completely restore optimal blood sugar balance and promote healthy blood lipid panels.

Fasting Mechanism: Ketosis

Your cells mainly run on energy generated from glucose or fatty acids. Ketosis is the state in which your cells are primarily being fueled by ATP generated from fatty acid metabolism in the form of ketones.

Ketosis quite literally means *fat-burning*.

The advantage of ketosis is that the energy generated from fats is much more stable and efficient than that of sugar. In fact, while in ketosis, blood sugar remains incredibly stable. It was likely this ability to enter ketosis that allowed our ancestors to survive periods of hardship when very little food was available.

Most people in modern times are constantly consuming foods and never enter ketosis. Instead they consistently have an abundance of glucose available for energy.

It is generally understood that the mechanism for inducing ketosis is a prolonged depletion of cellular glucose levels. This makes fasting the most efficient method of achieving the metabolic shift into ketosis.

Now let's break down why getting your body into ketosis might be a good idea.

Benefits of Ketosis

Many of the benefits from fasting may be a result of pushing the body into a state of ketosis.

Anti-Inflammatory

One of the primary mechanisms by which fasting and ketosis are thought to be beneficial for the body are that they are anti-inflammatory (20). This may be due to the fact that ketone metabolism creates a lower amount of oxidative stress compared to glucose metabolism.

Another potential reason for this may be the fact that fasting gives the digestive tract time to heal itself. Oftentimes poor diet, history of antibiotic use, or any number things can create a cascade of weak digestion. Weak digestion often leads to a higher susceptibility to microbiome imbalance, unwanted infections, and a massive amount of inflammation that affects the entire body.

I can say that in my clinical experience, fasting is incredible for healing inflammatory disorders stemming from gut issues.

Improvement in Metabolic Conditions

When we look at studies that compare carbohydrate restriction versus fat restriction, we see that restricting carbohydrates promotes much better outcomes in people with Type II Diabetes and heart disease (21).

In the journal *Current Nutrition Report* there was a review published in 2018 that investigated the efficacy of nutritional ketosis for weight loss and metabolic syndrome treatment (22). What they found was that inducing a state of ketosis improved just about every marker of metabolic health including: blood lipids, HbA1c (the insulin resistance marker we covered earlier), high-sensitivity CRP (a marker of inflammation), fasting insulin levels, blood sugar levels, and body fat.

Protection Against Neurodegenerative Diseases

A 2018 review published in the journal *Nature Reviews Neuroscience* concluded that cycles of positive and negative energy balance are optimal for brain health (23). An example of a positive energy state would be just after consuming a meal while a negative energy state would be fasting or exercise.

The authors of this study found that negative energy cycling:

- Improves cognition
- Enhances sensory-motor function
- Improves physical performance
- Promotes the growth of new neurons as a result of elevated ketone bodies
- Makes cells more resilient to stress
- Up-regulates neurotropic factor to enhance neuron growth

- Increases antioxidant defenses to protect brain cells against inflammation
- Promotes the growth of new mitochondria
- Promotes autophagy of weak and malfunctioning brain cells

In other words, fasting and ketosis are incredible for your brain. In fact, the authors also noted in this study that individuals who were eating 3 meals a day plus snacks were predisposed to suboptimal brain function, neurodegeneration, and psychiatric disorders!

What I thought was especially cool about this study was that there was not a specific fasting strategy that was ideal. As long as you regularly experience periods of negative energy balance you can obtain these benefits.

As we will cover later in this book, there are plenty of fasting strategies to choose from that can be suited to any lifestyle. All you have to do is simply choose one that makes sense for you!

Anxiolytic and Anti-Depressive Effects

The elevation of ketone bodies may have a stress-relieving effect in some humans. One study found that short-chain fatty acids and ketone bodies can regulate the nervous system through a protein-coupled receptor called GPR41 (24).

The authors of this study observed that under ketogenic conditions (when ketone bodies are elevated), there is a down-regulation of the sympathetic nervous system and slowing of the heart rate.

Another study published in 2019 separated a group of 1422 people in different fasting groups where they were assigned to fast for periods of 5, 10, 15, or 20 days (25). In addition to improvements in metabolic health, a massive 93.2% of participants reported an increase in physical and emotional well-being. THAT'S HUGE!

Anti-Cancer & Chemotherapy Booster

There are several studies which show an elevation of ketone bodies or short-chain fatty acids can inhibit cancer development. Additionally, there are studies in which fasting or ketogenesis are investigated for adjunct therapies alongside chemotherapy with promising results.

Generally speaking, as cancer progresses, cancer cells undergo something call the Warburg Effect. Here is what you need to know about the Warburg Effect: (26)

- Healthy cells either use the tricarboxylic acid (TCA) cycle or oxidative phosphorylation to make energy. They take glucose or ketone bodies out of the blood stream and generate ATP. This gives healthy cells the option to create energy from sugars or fats.

- Cancer Cells shift away from these processes and opt instead for a different one called glycolysis – which can ONLY use glucose

For this reason, many studies have suggested that depriving the body of glucose through fasting or ketogenic diet may be beneficial for treating cancer (27). A 2020 study piloted by one of the leading researchers in cancer metabolism, Thomas Seyfried, suggests that pushing the body into a ketogenic state may have a powerful role in breast cancer remission (28).

Another 2019 study, also piloted by Seyfried, suggests Ketogenic Metabolic Therapy should be considered as the new standard of care in certain cases of glioblastoma (29).

Finally, a review published in 2020 stated there is good evidence to suggest ketosis may be beneficial in treatment of prostate, colon, pancreas, and lung cancers when combined with traditional therapies (30). The study also concluded, however, that there is little evidence on whether ketosis is helpful for stomach and liver cancers.

Improvement in Mitochondrial Health

Since mitochondria are responsible for energy generation, they have a pivotal role in metabolic health. In fact, impaired mitochondrial function is involved in heart disease, diabetes, neurodegenerative disorders, and cancer.

A review of evidence cross-referencing the terms *ketosis* and *mitochondrial hormesis* found that inducing a state of ketosis is able to enhance mitochondrial function while also boosting antioxidant defense mechanisms (31).

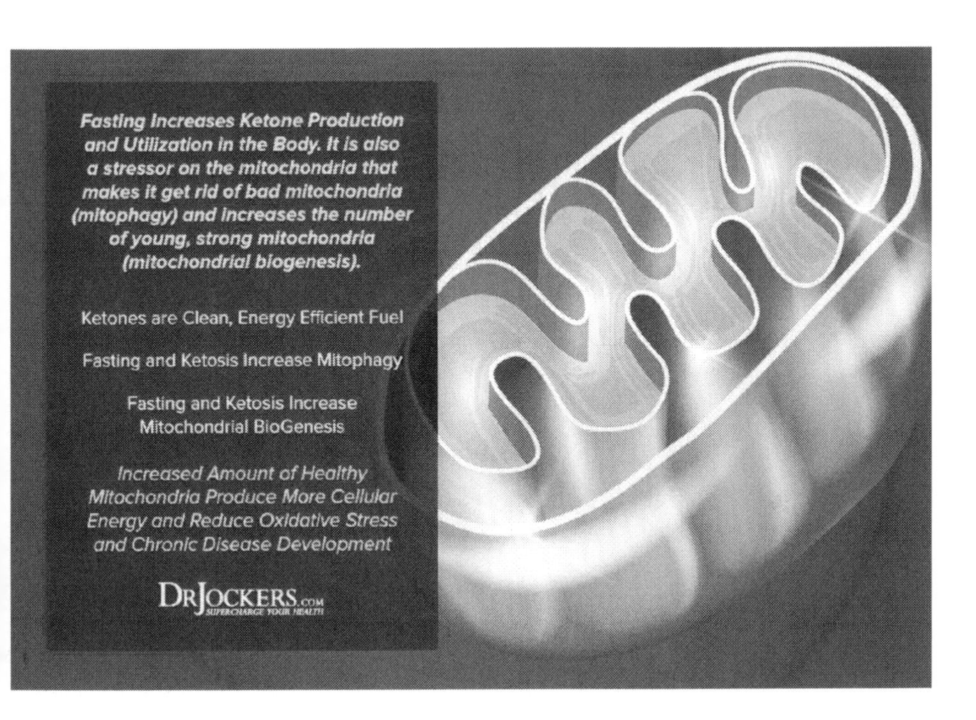

Fasting Mechanism: Increased Growth Hormone

Human growth hormone (HGH) is a hormone made by the master endocrine gland in your brain, the pituitary gland. HGH plays a major role in childhood development but it also keeps us physically young as we age. HGH also acts as a counter-regulatory hormone in fasting that prevents the body from going into starvation. In fact, every morning before you wake up your body will have a surge in growth hormone that helps raise your blood sugar and provide you with energy for the morning.

HGH is important for regulating muscle development, bone growth, immune activity, and metabolism. In fact, you may have seen commercials about HGH and how it is considered the ultimate anti-aging hormone. While these commercials usually try to sell you some expensive pill or cream, you can achieve optimal HGH levels without buying into these gimmicks.

Having optimal levels of HGH is also important for enhancing skin repair (reducing wrinkling), healing internal organs, protecting the brain against deterioration, and maintaining bone marrow production so that your body is able to make adequate red blood cells.

Unfortunately, HGH levels tend to decline with age.

After reaching 20 years of age, HGH tends to decline at a rate of 14% per decade. By the age of 40, HGH production has usually decreased by 30%. By the age of 60, HGH can decline by 80%!

This decline in HGH usually coincides with higher body fat, thinning and wrinkling of the skin, a weaker immune system, and a lower sex drive (32).

On top of age, other factors that negatively impact HGH include:

- Lack of exercise, especially resistance exercise
- Poor diet
- Insulin resistance
- Obesity
- Chronic stress
- Poor sleep

What Do You Do When HGH Plummets?

Well... As I mentioned earlier you could try hormone replacement therapy. One of the first HGH studies ever, published in the New England Journal of Medicine, found that after 6-months of receiving HGH they observed: (33)

- An 8lb muscle gain
- A 5.3 lb. fat loss
- Improved Skin Thickness

...And this is in men over 60 years old!

Another 2002 study published in the Journal of the American Medical Association found that these benefits extend to women as well (34)

This all sounds great but there is a pretty concerning issue: These individuals also had elevated blood sugar (some became pre-diabetic), increased fluid retention in tissues, elevated blood pressure, and the potential elevated risk for certain cancers.

Luckily, research suggests that the beneficial actions of HGH above can be enhanced through fasting – but with the opposite effect on blood sugar, blood pressure, and cancer risk (35, 36, 37, 38).

How Fasting Changes Growth Hormone

There are several studies that show significant increases in HGH in people who are fasting.

One study found that a 2-day fast stimulated a **5-fold increase in HGH** (39).

In fact, some research suggests that some of the most important benefits of fasting may come from HGH elevations. A 2014 study found that rats without growth hormone receptors (through genetic alteration) did not experience the same metabolic benefits of fasting as normal rats (40).

Another way to look at fasting and growth hormone are that it provides ideal conditions for growth hormone to stay at optimal levels.

What I mean by this is that things like high body-fat, high insulin levels, and frequent eating all lower growth hormone. Fasting helps to counteract the negative effects of each of these conditions so that HGH can do its thing.

For weight loss, the elevation in growth hormone may be advantageous for preserving muscle mass while losing body fat. In fact, some evidence suggests fasting preserves lean body mass during fat loss better than a calorically restricted diet.

For athletic performance, training in a fasted state may be the ultimate stimulus for muscle growth and fat loss. Although we still need studies done on this, there are an increasing number of athletes and bodybuilders who swear by training in a fasted state. Theoretically, the increased HGH levels during a workout should assist in muscle mass development and workout recovery.

There you have it, fasting provides a nice anti-aging boost of HGH but without all the negative affects you would get with hormone therapies!

Fasting Mechanism: AMPk

AMPk, also known as adenosine 5' monophosphate-activated protein kinase (don't worry – you don't have to memorize that), is an enzyme that plays a role in energy regulation of the cell. AMPk is something that all living organisms have preserved genetically. This means it probably played a really important role in our survival as a species!

Some scientists even go as far as saying that AMPk controls the aging process (41)

It works as a metabolic sensor, raising or lowering energy supply to cells. Primarily, when energy levels in the cell are low, AMPk pathways activate to raise them back up. AMPk does this by inhibiting energy-consuming processes and stimulating ATP production pathways (42).

Most notably, stressors that stimulate AMPk include caloric restriction, exercise, cold exposure, heat shock, fasting, and hypoxia (low oxygen levels).

Once AMPk is activated we see the following occur within the body:

- Increased fatty acid oxidation
- Increased insulin sensitivity
- Increased glucose uptake into muscles
- Promotion of ketosis
- Stimulation of mitochondrial biogenesis

These are, of course, all adaptations that occur with regular fasting.

A loss of AMPk signaling is associated with aging and may increase your risk of muscle loss and mitochondrial dysfunction (43).

AMPk seems like yet another great explanation for how fasting has been shown to extend lifespan in just about every animal it's been tested on!

Fasting Mechanism: Stem Cells

The final major fasting mechanism of benefit I want to discuss is the up-regulation of stem cells.

A stem cell is a cell that has not yet been assigned a function in the body. It can become a liver cell or a bone cell (or anything else) at any given moment depending on the demands of the body. Once a cell changes from a stem cell into something else, it stays that way until the body eventually breaks it down to make room for new cells.

If the pathways that regulate stem cells are not operating properly, there is a higher risk of cancer and accelerated aging (44, 45).

This is how organs regenerate and stay healthy. Through autophagy (breaking down old cells) and through proliferation of stem cells that are able to replace those old cells.

So, if theoretically you could speed up autophagy and stem cell production – you could heal the body much more quickly right?

Do you know what does both of these things exceptionally well? FASTING

Perhaps this is an explanation for people who are able to bounce back from some pretty serious conditions by fasting!

We have had evidence for years that fasting extends life span in certain types of yeast and many different animals. We've also seen that fasting promotes stem cell generation, rejuvenates the immune system, slows down bone loss with age, promotes brain growth in the hippocampus, and improves cognitive performance in mice (46).

Do these benefits also transfer to humans?

Well, one study took a look at this.

A study published in *Current Stem Cell Reports* compared Caloric Restriction, Fasting, High-fat Diets, and Ketogenic Diets and their respective effects on the regulation of stem cells (47).

In the study the authors noted that, while fasting and caloric restriction both provide a longer health span and life span, fasting provides unique benefits that suggest fasting boosts stem cell function. These include:

- Increased stress resistance of DNA against damage
- Protection against chemotherapy side effects
- Reversing age-related degeneration

This study summarized recent findings that fasting can boost the following types of stem cells:

- Intestine
- Skeletal Muscle
- Blood Cell Forming Cells in the bone marrow

This study also noted fasting benefits for protection against neurodegenerative disorders.

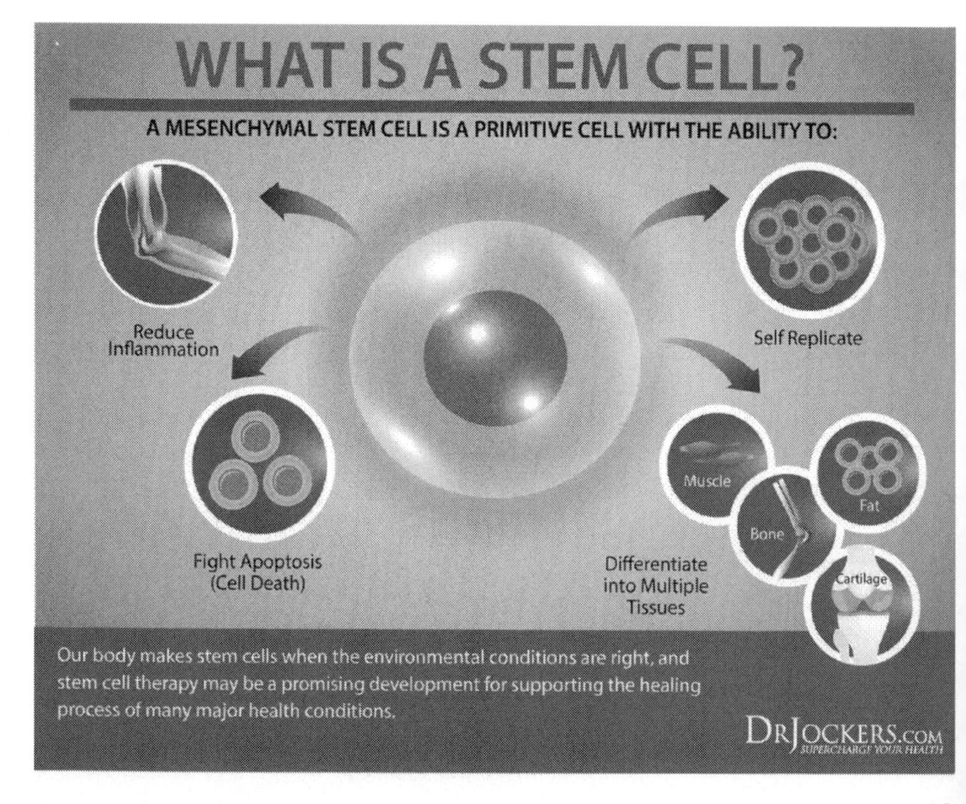

The Synergy of Benefits

In this chapter we've taken quite the deep dive into some science and 5 major reasons why fasting is so great for you:

1. Insulin sensitivity
2. Ketosis
3. Growth Hormone
4. AMPk
5. Stem Cells

Taken altogether, you can see how fasting is a powerhouse for health. You don't need to spend ridiculous amounts of money on fancy foods, supplements, labs, and everything else.

Can these things be helpful? Absolutely. I have my own brand of pharmaceutical grade supplements, I have a lab-ordering portal on my site, and nutrition is important! I even have a fasting support supplement stack that I use. I'm not saying that fasting will solve every problem ever... But it is by far and away the most powerful strategy most people can start with.

Chapter 3: Fasting Myths

Ever told someone you were thinking about trying fasting? It's a HUGE deal, right? Like everyone who loves and cares about you just freaks out with concern that you're about to do something terrible?

"You're going to starve yourself?!"

"Why don't you just exercise more and stop trying to do all these drastic things?!"

"You're going to develop an eating disorder!"

"Fasting doesn't work! You'll just gain all the weight back when it's over!"

"You're going to be so miserable!"

It's interesting... You can eat junk food all day. Drink beer. Lose sleep staying up watching TV night after night... and no one second guesses it. These are normal things.

...But the second you tell someone you're going too fast for your health; they think you've gone mad! Why is that??

Even though fasting has a rich history and strong scientific support, it seems there are strong myths behind this idea of purposefully abstaining from food.

Let's break down some of the most pervasive fasting myths.

Fasting Myth: It is Unnatural and Unhealthy for the Body

This is the most prominent fasting myth of all. Although we pretty much addressed this myth by going through the history and science of fasting – let's dissect it once more.

Think back to what you have likely been taught about nutrition since you were a child. The first nutrition resource we were all exposed to was the United States Dietary Association (USDA) guidelines. While the way they have presented their recommendations has changed over the years, the food pyramid seems to be the one everyone remembers well. You know, the one that essentially said you could eat as much bread, cereal, and pasta as you want – but also make sure you eat your fruits and vegetables... then a little bit of meat and fat to top it off.

These are hardly good practices for optimal health.

You've also likely heard that eating 3-5 meals throughout the day is the best way to keep your blood sugar balanced and metabolism high. I believe this is one of the main reasons people think fasting is bad.

In my experience, I can say that following this recommendation more often than not actually leads to weight gain, sugar cravings, and mood imbalances. This is because insulin was never meant be spiked several times a day.

The more frequently your insulin is stimulated throughout the day, the more likely you are to pack on body fat.

As we discussed in Chapter 2, fasting has the reverse effect on insulin levels.

In addition, I should reiterate that fasting also:

- Promotes mitochondrial health
- Assists DNA repair
- Accelerates autophagy and stem-cell production
- Stimulates Fat Burning
- And has been a part of our survival since humans existed

It is not unnatural or unhealthy in the slightest!

Fasting Myth: It Slows Down Your Metabolism

Another myth that persists from the USDA recommendations we were all raised believing. Eating multiple times a day does NOT make you a better fat burner. In fact, it much more likely to promote fat storage. This goes especially if your meals are heavy in carbohydrates or you are a particularly sedentary individual.

Like we discussed in Chapter 2, fasting promotes ketosis and a significant surge in growth hormone levels. These two effects are fantastic for your metabolism as well as burning fat and building lean muscle.

What DOES slow down the metabolism is not eating enough for a prolonged period of time. This is why traditional dietary approaches may not always be so successful.

By using an online tool or health tracking device, you can determine your baseline metabolic needs and ensure you are eating enough calories.

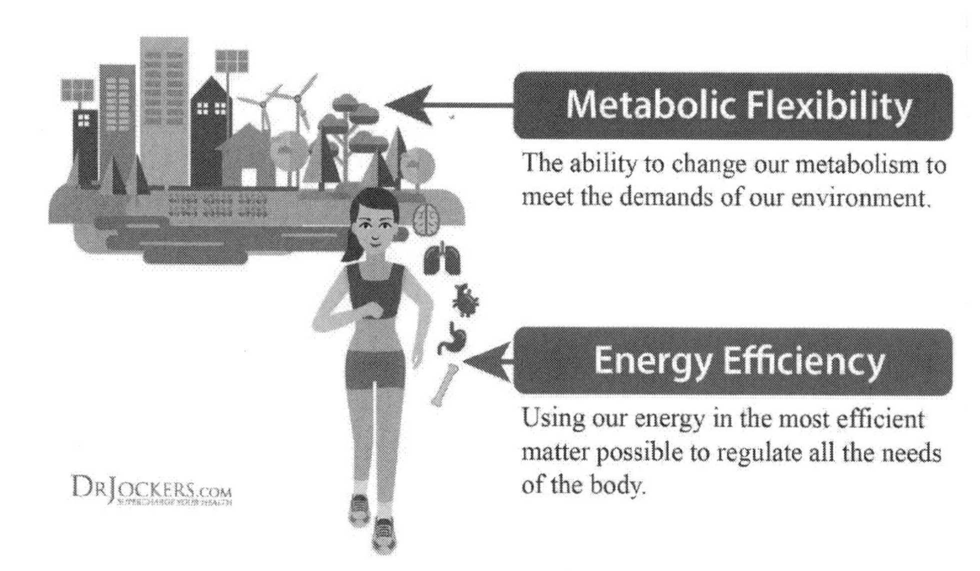

Fasting Myth: It Causes Nutrient Deficiencies

Nutrient deficiencies are real, and they can be a huge problem.

Here is a list of some of the most common reasons for nutrient deficiencies:

1. A diet low in nutrients (DUH)
2. Poor digestion due to low stomach acid levels
3. Leaky gut, due to chronic inflammation of the intestinal lining
4. Blood sugar imbalances, preventing insulin from transporting nutrients into the cell

5. Chronic stress

Fasting will not cause nutrient deficiencies unless the foods you are eating are lacking in nutrients. In fact, fasting can actually resolve poor digestion, leaky gut, and blood sugar imbalances – making you BETTER at absorbing nutrients.

So then, all you have to do to prevent nutrient deficiencies while fasting is eat nutrient-dense foods!

Here's my quick rundown of a nutrient-dense diet:

Remove inflammatory foods like refined sugar and most grains. This means no bread, pastas, sugary drinks, or junk foods.

You also want to avoid vegetable oils like the plague. There is no place for oils like canola, safflower, corn, cottonseed or soybean in the human diet. They are highly inflammatory.

Base your diet on pasture-raised or wild caught whole animal foods like muscle meat, organs, bone broths, and butter. These should be base of every meal. Then add in organic fruits and vegetables.

If you want additional micronutrient support, consider a multivitamin or a grass-fed beef liver supplement.

Fasting Myth: It Causes Muscle Loss

This myth comes from the fitness industry. Bodybuilders and fitness enthusiasts alike are well known for promoting a 6-meal-a-day eating plan to prevent muscle loss and burn fat.

The truth is, fasting is probably ideal for physique. As long as you eat enough calories and optimize your protein intake, fasting promotes the ideal hormonal conditions for building muscle and burning fat at the same time.

As we discussed in Chapter 2, fasting promotes ketosis and a rise in growth hormone.

Shifting into fasting-induced ketosis will mobilize fat stores in the body to be burned as energy. Simultaneously, high growth hormone levels will promote muscle growth.

A recent study confirmed this idea (1). Over an 8-week period, body fat and muscle mass were monitored in two groups: an alternate-day fasting group and a non-fasting group. This study found that after 8 weeks, the fasting group lost 12 lbs. of fat with no significant loss in muscle mass.

Using an online caloric intake calculator will help you determine the ideal number of calories and protein you need. When these are optimized, you will likely be able to burn fat and build muscle at the same time.

Fasting Myth: Fasting is an Eating Disorder (Or Causes Them)

It is not likely that fasting would cause an eating disorder. It is possible, however, that a dietary strategy that has been promoted for weight loss would attract someone who already struggles with an eating disorder.

Talking about fasting and eating disorders exposes a fine line in how we think about dietary decisions.

Yes, eating too much can be considered an eating disorder.

Yes, eating too little can be considered an eating disorder.

Each of these can have very serious consequences and should not be taken lightly.

When it comes down to it, the reason you are partaking in a dietary strategy can make all the difference.

Don't aim to lose weight. Aim to get healthy.

Calculate your dietary needs and fit them into your fasting routine. Fasting this way will optimize your hormones and energy levels so that your body can settle on an ideal weight in the process.

If you are someone who has struggled with disordered eating I recommend easing into intermittent fasting. Starting with just 12-hour fasts and ensuring you are getting adequate nutrition.

It can also help to have an accountability partner that is close to you and understands the eating disorder patterns you have struggled with. This way they can help you stay on track if you begin to fall back into disordered eating patterns.

Fasting Myth: It is Dangerous for People with Diabetes

For Pre-Diabetics and Type 2 Diabetics

I have had many diabetics come to me with concern about fasting and low blood sugar. While this is a valid concern, it is not something to stop you from fasting.

In the case of prediabetes or Type II diabetes, we discussed in chapter 2 how fasting can actually help reverse these conditions by restoring insulin sensitivity. On the other hand, the conventional recommendation to eat frequently throughout the day can actually make insulin sensitivity worse.

One study published in the *World Journal of Diabetes* reaffirms this idea by showing that intermittent fasting improved weight loss, fasting blood sugar, and helped stabilize blood sugar after dinner in a group of type 2 diabetics (2).

Another review study published in March 2020 in *Current Diabetes Reports* concluded that there is no increased risk of hypoglycemia in type 2 diabetics. In fact, they mention case studies in which type 2 diabetes has been reversed using fasting methods (3).

For Type I Diabetics

Type I diabetics who cannot produce their own insulin will need to closely monitor their blood sugar if they are to attempt fasting. These individuals may still be able to fast for 12 to 16 hours depending on the stability of their blood sugar levels.

Blood sugar and energy levels will be your gauge for when it is time to re-feed.

****Note: If you have diabetes or any other medical condition, it is always advisable to discuss intermittent fasting or any other diet changes with your healthcare practitioner who understands your unique health history.**

Fasting Myth: It Causes Binge Eating

Two things that largely dictate our hunger and eating behaviors are a hormone called leptin, and blood sugar levels.

Leptin is a hormone that signals to your brain when you should stop eating – or when you have achieved satiety (a sense of fullness).

The more insulin resistant someone is, the more likely they are to be leptin resistant as well. This leads to chronic hunger even though the body has consumed more than enough calories... and the fat just piles on.

This makes blood sugar levels and leptin resistance equally tied to hunger and uncontrollable eating behaviors.

Fasting may effective for resetting leptin signaling and should therefore improve your ability to control the urge to binge eat.

In my experience, many people report that fasting for a period of 48 hours or longer is the most effective for preventing binge eating. This seems to be a sweet spot for resetting the bodies hunger signaling and most people simply find it difficult to binge eat because they achieve satiation much more quickly.

Another helpful strategy is to consume satiating foods that pack a lot of nutrition.

Some of the best satiating foods to eat when you break an intermittent fast include:

- Eggs
- Grass Fed Red Meat (Especially Fatty Cuts)

- Wild Caught Fish
- Grass Fed Dairy (If you tolerate dairy)
- Saturated Fats (Butter, Coconut Oil)
- Organ Meats
- Soups or Stews Made with Bone Broth
- Avocados and Avocado Oil
- Coconut Milk and Coconut Oil
- Olives and Olive Oil
- Fruits, Especially Berries, Lemons & Limes.
- Artichokes & Asparagus
- Cruciferous Veggies (Broccoli, Cauliflower, etc.)
- Dark Green Leafy Veggies
- Sweet Potatoes
- Sprouted and/or Soaked Grains, Beans, Lentils, Nuts, and Seeds
- Nut Butters
- Vegetable Soup

****Note: The foods above are specifically for breaking fasts shorter than 48 hours. Fasts longer than 48 hours will cause the digestive system to down-regulate itself and will need gradual reintroduction of easy to digest foods. We will discuss how to do this later in this book.**

If you want to make delicious meals out of the ingredients listed above, check the recipe section of my website – drjockers.com. Every recipe is blood-sugar friendly and nutritious, considers both omnivorous and plant-based diets, and there may even be some delicious cookie recipes (wink-wink).

Making fasting a regular practice and building your discipline will also help to control impulses over time and can be an excellent tool for breaking addictive behaviors altogether!

Fasting Myth: You Shouldn't Exercise While Fasting

Exercise might actually be <u>one of the best</u> things you can do while fasting. While this may not hold true for everyone, fasted exercise can be a great way to boost fat burning and lose weight.

This can be a great benefit if you have weight to lose.

If you are an otherwise healthy individual looking to optimize hormones and muscle mass, you can use this method as well. The nuance for lean individuals will be ensuring that they consume adequate calories and protein during the re-feed window following exercise.

As we discussed previously in this chapter, fasting is unlikely to lead to muscle loss unless you do not eat enough in your re-feeding window.

Considering fasting creates an anabolic (growth promoting) surge in growth hormone while also stimulating fat-burning, it can be a great combination with resistance exercise. Studies suggest that endurance-based activities may not go so well with fasting, however (4).

Ultimately, you will need to determine for yourself whether or not you perform better in your specific fitness routine while fasted or not.

I personally perform intense fasted resistance training sessions 2-4 times per week and feel that this is when I am able to perform my best.

Fasted Exercise Hack: Sometimes I will use an exogenous ketone supplement before my workouts when I need an extra boost. It is a great stimulant-free pre-workout.

Fasting Myth: It Will Make You Feel Hangry

You know that feeling when you miss a meal and suddenly everyone around you just bugs the crap out of you? You know... that hangry feeling?

This happens when someone who is not adapted to fasting experiences a drop in blood sugar. They become tired, hungry, and irritable.

When you first begin fasting you may experience some energy dips. As you continue, however, fasting will become second nature.

Most people report that, while the first 1 or 2 fasts are a little uncomfortable, afterwards they become accustomed to it and actually feel very energized while fasting. It is a little like starting an exercise routine for the first time. The first few days are the most difficult part but once it is a routine it's enjoyable!

So, this myth isn't entirely untrue... but it is not something you will have to deal with forever I promise.

The quickest way to get past this feeling is too fast for 48 hours or more. This is the fast and slightly more uncomfortable route to beginning fasting.

You can also ease your way into longer fasts by beginning with a ketogenic nutrition plan and gradually building up your fasting periods.

We will dive deeper into fasting implementation later in this book.

Fasting Myth: It Will Cause Food Cravings

Partially true, but not entirely.

Just like feeling hangry, cravings will likely be stronger in the beginning – yet diminish with time.

If you need some strategies to ward off cravings, try some of these:

- **Have black coffee**
- **Start your day with a butter coffee (this would technically break the fast but maintain ketosis)**
- **Sparkling Mineral Water**
- **Go for a 10-minute walk or run**

Time to Implement!

So far, we have deeply investigated the origins and science behind fasting. At this point you have likely decided whether or not you are going to try it or not.

Maybe you already fast but you want to do it with more intention. Either way, it is time to learn the strategies.

In the following chapters we are going to dive into how fasting strategies based on length and health goals.

Chapter 4: Intermittent Fasting Strategies

This chapter on intermittent fasting strategies will strictly focus on fasts that are employed on a daily basis. There are 6 main fasting strategies that are programmed on a daily cycle:

- **Simple Fast:** 12 Hours
- **Brunch Fast**: 14 Hours
- **Crescendo Fast**: 16 Hours – 2 days out of the week
- **Cycle Fast**: 16 Hours – 3 days out of the week
- **Strong Fast**: 16-18 Hours
- **Warrior Fast (Sometimes referred to as OMAD or, One Meal a Day)**: 19-21 Hours

Keep in mind that there are ultimately an infinite number of ways you can employ fasting. The strategies below are a simple way to get started and work your way into more advanced strategies that I have been using clinically for over a decade.

As the book continues, we will cover more nuanced versions of fasting or "fasting-mimicking" diets that can be used for your unique situation.

Simple Fast

A simple fast is a 12-hour fast. Typically, the majority of a simple fast is done while sleeping – making it a great starting point for someone getting into fasting. If you are someone who is intimidated by fasting, start here and you'll likely soon realize that you are very capable of adopting some type of fasting routine.

Keep in mind that not everyone will feel great fasting 21 hours a day or a 5-day water fast. That is okay. You need to test different strategies out and find what works best for your goals and lifestyle.

Even a simple 12-hour fast can:

- Help improve sleep and overnight healing
- Improve liver function to detoxify the body
- Improve food cravings and addictions
- Stimulate fat burning
- Help heal the lining of the gut

A 12-hour fast means you are left with a 12-hour eating window. This makes it very straight-forward when planning into your current routine.
If you finish dinner at 6pm, eat breakfast at 6am.

If you finish dinner at 8pm, eat breakfast at 8am.

Simple.

Here's some tips on how I would plan it:

Determine your preferred bedtime - I personally like to be in bed by 10PM

Finish your last meal of the day 3-4 hours before bed for optimal digestion – This would mean I need to try and finish dinner by 6 or 7pm.

Then fast for 12 hours!

This would mean I can eat again at about 6 or 7 am. Easy.

A simple fast is a good time to start a morning hydration routine. When you wake up, drink 8–16oz of water. Adding a high-quality electrolyte powder that does not have any calories can help.

Most people will find that this type of fast is no problem. If you find that this is the case, try extending the fasting window by two hours and making it a brunch fast instead.

It would be a good idea to spend about 2 weeks on each fasting style to ensure you are able to do it consistently with no issues.

Brunch Fast

A brunch fast is 14 hours.

So, in the example above: If you finish dinner at 6pm, then you can eat breakfast at 8am

If you finish dinner at 8pm, you eat breakfast at 10am.

Technically, it takes about 12 hours for your body to process your last meal and truly enter a fasted state. This is when most people will switch on fat-burning.

Although a brunch fast is only 2 hours longer than a simple fast, this gives your body a chance to truly adapt to burning fat for energy. This is the beginning of a metabolic shift that makes your body energy efficient and less reliant on constantly consuming food.

A brunch fast is great for people who have to start work early in the morning or who like to exercise when they wake up.

For the average person, the optimal eating window would likely be somewhere around 8am to 6pm to allow for complete digestion before sleep.

If you are someone who tends to have a late dinner (after 7pm or within 2 hours of bed), then a crescendo or cycle fast may suit your lifestyle a little better.

Crescendo Fast

A crescendo fast is a 16-hour fast performed only twice per week, on non-consecutive days.

The jump from a 14-hour fast to a 16-hour fast is quite significant metabolically. It is more challenging on the body, yet provides some improved benefits like more fat-burning and better insulin sensitivity.

Instead of jumping right into a 16-hour fast every day, a crescendo fast is performed only 2 times per week.

This is a great option for people with unpredictable schedules, those who feel comfortable doing the brunch fast, and lean, active females in particular.

Female physiology can be very sensitive to fasting or caloric restriction. Many females find that if they fast too strictly for their body type, there can sometimes be hormonal changes that lead to irregular periods, amenorrhea, infertility, bone density changes, and reduction in ovary size (1, 2, 3, 4).

This is because of a gland in the brain called the hypothalamus that regulates the release of reproductive hormones gonadotropin-releasing hormone (GnRH), follicle stimulating hormone (FSH), and luteinizing hormone (LH).

This hormone pathway is designed to prepare the female body for pregnancy. When the hypothalamus senses an energy deficit in a woman with a low body fat %, it will begin to shift towards 'survival mode'. This basically means the hypothalamus will begin to shut down energy demanding processes – in this case growing a fetus – in order to keep you healthy.

This makes crescendo fasting one of the most optimal fasting strategies for women who are already low in body fat and live a very active lifestyle with a lot of stressors. For these individuals, crescendo fasting allows for greater fasting benefits without the potential negative side effects.

To plan a crescendo fast, you will pick 2 non-consecutive days out of the week to perform a 16-hour fast. For example, you could choose Monday and Wednesday or Sunday and Thursday. You can pick any two days that fit your lifestyle and are not back-to-back.

After you choose your days, applying the 16-hour fast will leave you with an 8-hour eating window. Deciding if you'd like this eating window in the morning or afternoon depends on your goals.

Many people prefer to fast in the mornings as it provides them with heightened mental clarity and focus. Also, many people start work early in the morning and they'd rather not have to wake up earlier to make breakfast.

On the other hand, eating in the morning may act as a circadian cue which may help you get deeper sleep at night and promote weight loss (5). Some people simply like to enjoy dinner with their family – so they eat later in the day. There are many different reasons to choose a morning or evening feeding window.

The most important thing is to extend your fasting schedule gradually over time and listen to your body. Once you feel comfortable with a crescendo fast you can add one more non-consecutive fasting day to make it a cycle fast.

Cycle Fast

A cycle fast is a 16-hour fast performed ***3 times per week***, on non-consecutive days. It is a crescendo fast, plus one more fasting day.

For example, you could fast Monday, Wednesday, Friday or Sunday, Tuesday, Thursday.

This is a logical progression from a crescendo fast and working up to a daily 16-hour fast, if that is a goal of yours.

As you can imagine, crescendo and cycle fasting will require a bit more planning compared to simple or brunch fasting.

The key is to plan ahead and know what daily activities are going to be planned around being in a fasted state or a fed state. Think about things like work schedules, exercise planning, travel, and social gatherings you have planned.

Strong Fast

A strong fast is a 16 to 18-hour fast.

If you finish dinner at 6pm, you will not eat again until 10 am or 12pm the next day – depending on if you are fasting closer to 16 or 18 hours.
This is the sweet spot in which many people feel they derive the most benefits from fasting. If you are fasting to assist with healing from a particular health issue, regular 16-hour fasts would be a great goal to shoot for.

This is the fasting strategy I follow personally most days, saving all my meals for a 6 to 8-hour window in the afternoon when I spend time with my family. I also tend to eat ketogenic on most days as I discuss in detail in my book Keto Metabolic Breakthrough.

Once you have been fasting for some time and have worked your way up to a strong fast, this is when your body will likely enter a state of mild ketosis every day.

As we discussed in Chapter 2, having elevated levels of ketones in the body has many benefits like keeping your brain healthy, lifting your mood, and reducing inflammation.

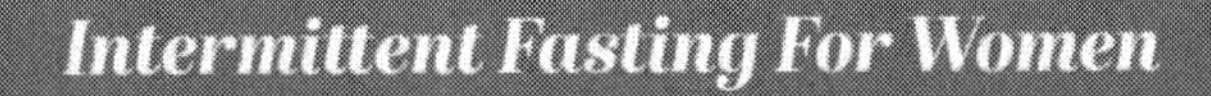

Women can get great benefits from intermittent fasting but they need to be cautious as they get started in order to prevent hormonal dysfunction.

BENEFITS OF INTERMITTENT FASTING

- Reduces Inflammation and and Improves Fat Burning
- Improves Metabolic Flexibility, Mental Health and Energy Levels
- Anti-Aging Benefits for Skin, Joints and Complexion

KEY CONSIDERATIONS TO REMEMBER

- Women Tend to Have a More Sensitive Stress Response than Men
- Fertility Hormones May Be Sensitive to Longer Periods without Food and Nutrients
- Hunger and Satiety Hormones May Be Impacted Negatively

INITIAL FASTING STRATEGIES TO APPLY

- ***Simple Fast*** - 12 Hours Overnight Between Meals Daily
- ***Brunch Fast*** - 14 Hours Overnight Between Meals Daily
- ***Crescendo Fasting*** - 16 Hours Overnight Between Meals 2 Days Per Week.

If you feel good with these, you can continue to progress the intensity of the fast where you would increase either the amount of time fasting or the frequency

CHECK POINTS

- Monitor How You Are Feeling on a Daily and Weekly Basis
- Make Sure You Aren't Overwhelming Your Body with Stress

REASONS TO REDUCE THE INTENSITY OF THE FAST

Energy Drops
Brain Fog
Major Mood Swings
Insomnia
Feel Cold All the Time
Hair Loss
Heart Arrhythmia
Menstrual Irregularities

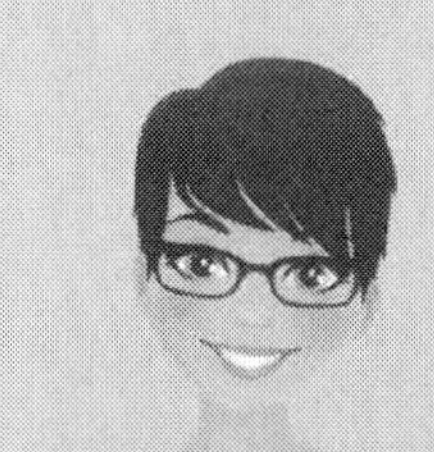

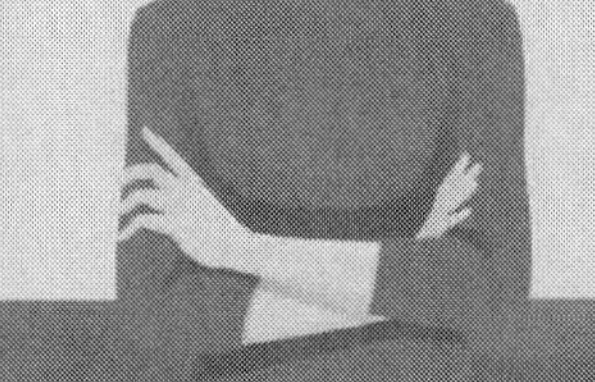

DRJOCKERS.COM

Warrior Fast and OMAD

A warrior fast is a 19 to 21-hour fast.

The warrior fast is an advanced intermittent fasting strategy being that it is the longest.

OMAD, or One Meal a Day, takes the warrior fast even further in that it specifies a 23-hour fast with only a 1-hour eating window.

While warrior fasting or OMAD likely provide the highest fat-burning and autophagy benefits, this method is for people who have already comfortably completed daily strong fasts and have even implemented periodic 24-hour fasting periods for several weeks or even months with no issues.

To perform a warrior fast, if you finish dinner at 6pm, you would eat again between 1 and 3pm the next day with only a 3–5 hour eating window.

For OMAD, you would simply choose a 1-hour eating window (such as 5 to 6pm) and fast outside of that window.

It is extremely important to consider your caloric needs while performing these longer fasts. For OMAD in particular, you will generally need to eat a very large amount of food to ensure you are getting adequate nutrition.

Chapter 5: Weekly & Extended Fasting Strategies

This chapter will focus on weekly and extended fasting strategies.

There are 6 approaches detailed in this chapter:

- **One Day a Week:** One 24-hour fast per week
- **5:2 Fasting:** 24-hour modified or pure fast, 2 days out of the week
- **4:3 Fasting:** 24-hour modified or pure fast, 3 days out of the week
- **Alternate-Day Fasting:** 24-hour fast, every other day
- **Rolling 48-Hour Fasting:** One meal every 48 hours
- **Extended Day Fasting:** 3–5 day fast (or more), typically performed on occasion

You will likely notice that some of these strategies are similar to the intermittent fasting strategies discussed in Chapter 4. The main difference in the weekly fasting strategies is that they involve a 24-hour fast (or multiple), employed on a weekly rhythm.

One Day a Week

A 24-hour fast performed once per week is one of the best beginner strategies for fasting. It is also very practical. While not everyone can tolerate a daily 16-hour fast, the vast majority of people can handle one 24-hour fast per week just fine.

Performing a 24-hour fast is also great for gaining the benefits of autophagy without having to disrupt your current lifestyle too much. This allows you to maintain relatively normal eating windows on most days, while still getting some of the benefits of fasting.

The best way to implement a 24-hour fast is to choose the day of the week with the lowest demands. For example, most people find that fasting from Saturday night dinner to Sunday night dinner works very well.

A 24-hour fast can also be combined with intermittent fasting and cyclical eating.

A popular weekly cycle that I recommend is:

Monday–Friday: 16-hour intermittent fast with Ketogenic Meals
Saturday: 16-hour fast with a higher carbohydrate reefed
Sunday: 24-hour fast

This is where you can play around with different fasting time windows and styles of eating to see what your body responds best to. Some people do better with carbs while others prefer ketogenic eating. Some people like to maintain a plant-based eating template while others like the combination of fasting and carnivore nutrition. Each of these strategies have an application!

We'll discuss how these combinations can be used in Chapter 7 – Fasting for Chronic Disease.

5:2 Fasting

A 5:2 fast is a 24-hour fast, performed twice per week. These 24-hour fasts are performed on non-consecutive days.

The 5:2 strategy can also be employed as a modified fast where the 2 days you choose as fasting days are actually caloric restriction days. On these days, instead of avoiding food altogether, you can consume a small meal of 500 calories for women and 600 calories for men.

An example of a weekly 5:2 rhythm would be fasting on Monday and Thursday, while each other day is a normal eating day. This allows for 2–3 days between each 24-hour fast.

This specific 5:2 modified fast has been researched and found to improve insulin sensitivity and reduce body fat (1).

My personal weekly routine resembles the 5:2 protocol. I perform 24-hour fasts on Wednesday and Saturday. I perform about a 16-hour fast on every other day with low-carb or ketogenic meals. On Sundays I feast and consume more carbs. This is the complete protocol that makes me feel my best.

4:3 Fasting

Naturally, if you scale up from a 5:2 fast, you could add an additional fasting day to your weekly schedule. Again, you would want these to be non-consecutive days.

For example, your weekly 4:3 fasting schedule could look something like this:

- Monday: Fast
- Tuesday: Normal Eating
- Wednesday: Fast
- Thursday: Normal Eating
- Friday: Fast
- Saturday & Sunday: Normal Eating

Typically, it is recommended that, on fasting days, you adhere strictly to the fast. On normal eating days you would want to eat in a way that does not feel restricted so that you can achieve satiety and no feel pressured to eat junk foods.

To reiterate from Chapter 4, foods you want to focus on for maximum benefits are nutrient-dense and filling such as:

- **Eggs**
- **Grass Fed Red Meat (Especially Fatty Cuts)**
- **Wild Caught Fish**
- **Grass Fed Dairy (If you tolerate dairy)**
- **Saturated Fats (Butter, Coconut Oil)**
- **Organ Meats**
- **Soups or Stews Made with Bone Broth**
- **Avocados and Avocado Oil**
- **Coconut Milk and Coconut Oil**
- **Olives and Olive Oil**
- **Fruits, Especially Berries, Lemons & Limes.**

- **Artichokes & Asparagus**
- **Cruciferous Veggies (Broccoli, Cauliflower, etc.)**
- **Dark Green Leafy Veggies**
- **Sweet Potatoes**
- **Sprouted and/or Soaked Grains, Beans, Lentils, Nuts, and Seeds**
- **Nut Butters**
- **Vegetable Soup**

In cases like this I like to give this simple advice: eat nutrient-dense foods to the point of satisfaction as to prevent the temptation for snacks.

Protein and fat are your friends here. In fact, many people find that following a mostly ketogenic meal template makes fasting days fairly easy to adhere to. This is something you may consider trying out for yourself.

Alternate-Day Fasting

Alternate-day fasting Is pretty much self-explanatory. You eat normally one day, then fast the next. You repeat this pattern indefinitely until your health goals change or you feel that you need to increase or decrease the amount of time you fast.

Alternate-day fasting is one of the more heavily researched fasting structures.

A recent 2020 review published in the American Journal of Medicine suggested that alternate-day fasting may be an effective dietary strategy for reducing your risk of heart disease (2). The authors propose that this reduction of heart disease risk is likely related to improvements in weight, blood pressure, cholesterol, and blood sugar control.

A clinical trial published in 2019 compared the effects of alternate-day fasting to traditional caloric restriction with some pretty cool results. The authors of this study concluded that alternate-day fasting may actually be more effective than traditional dieting for losing weight, lowering blood pressure, and improving blood sugar control (3).

Finally, another recent study suggested that alternate-day fasting may help slow tumor progression in subjects undergoing cancer treatment (4). This approach seems to be further supported with a ketogenic eating plan. This is likely due to the observation that, in many types of cancer, cancer cells have an impaired metabolism that makes them less effective at using ketones for energy (5).

We will discuss the specifics of fasting in the midst of cancer later in this book.

Rolling 48-hour Fasts

Rolling 48-hour fasts are an advanced fasting strategy that should only be followed with close supervision. On this schedule you only consume one meal every 48-hours.

While there is no research specific to this fasting plan, there are hundreds of anecdotal success stories following this plan. In most cases these are very obese individuals who are attempting accelerated weight loss or individuals healing from specific diseases that have not responded to other therapies.

With such an intense fasting routine, it would be very important to track water intake and keep electrolyte levels balanced.

This would mean consuming an electrolyte solution containing the recommended daily allowance (RDA) amounts of sodium, magnesium, and potassium throughout the day to keep intracellular hydration balanced.

The electrolyte RDAs for adults are:

Sodium: 1500mg (studies show that 5000 mg is likely what you want to shoot for) (6)
Potassium: 4700mg
Magnesium: 300–500mg

Most pre-made electrolyte brands contain either sugar or artificial sweetener. While stevia is a natural sweetener, even just the sweet taste can promote cravings during a fast. That means you will need to make your own without any sweetener.

Here is a homemade fasting electrolyte solution recipe you can use:

Mixed in 1 Liter of Water,

Sea Salt – ½–1 tsp (providing about 1000 mg of sodium)
Potassium chloride – ½ tsp (providing about 1600 mg of potassium)
Magnesium Glycinate – ½ tsp (providing about 200 mg of magnesium)

You would want to slowly sip on this solution throughout the day. If you are urinating very frequently or have loose bowels, then that is a sign to back off or drink plain water temporarily.

To reach the RDA amounts of each of these electrolytes, you would need to drink approximately 3 Liters of this solution.

Each of these ingredients are cheap and easy to find. Sea salt and potassium chloride (marketed as a salt replacement) can usually be found at the grocery store while magnesium glycinate powder will be found online.

Staying hydrated during longer fasts is critical for maintaining energy levels and preventing the rare (yet dangerous) condition called re-feeding syndrome. We will discuss this more in-depth in the Troubleshooting Fasting Challenges Chapter.

Extended-Day Fasting

Any fast 48-hours or longer is considered an extended fast.

Research suggests that performing a 5-day fast once a month for three months in a row is an effective strategy for reducing risk factors for diabetes, cancer, heart disease, and the effects of aging (7).

In my experience, extended fasting is a powerful intervention for those with cancer, metabolic disease, autoimmunity, and diseases of the digestive tract.

The length of an extended fast is highly dependent on your current health state. The longest fast ever recorded was 382 days. This was a 27-year-old male who initially weighed 456 pounds and completed his fast at a weight of 180 pounds. That's incredible!

Even after 5 years, this man maintained his weight loss with no side effects from the massive fast.

Obviously, not everyone is suited to perform such a fast. In this case, there was close medical supervision and administration of vitamins to retain optimal nutrition status within the body.

What this story does show us though, is that the body is well-suited for fasting. Most individuals can complete a 3–5 day fast with some planning. The biggest barrier to completing an extended fast is a mental barrier.

During an extended fast, you will want to keep stress levels low, hydrate diligently (refer to the guidelines just above), and closely monitor yourself for negative side effects.

While the longest I have ever fasted is 5 days, I do know several people who have achieved great results fasting for longer than 5 days. Approach this territory cautiously and consult your doctor before jumping into an extended fast. There are fasting centers located around the world who specialize in supervising extended fasts as well.

While extended fasting is the most advanced strategy in this book, I have seen it transform lives. This is why there are 2 full chapters dedicated to how to prepare for and execute an extended fast for maximum benefits coming up.

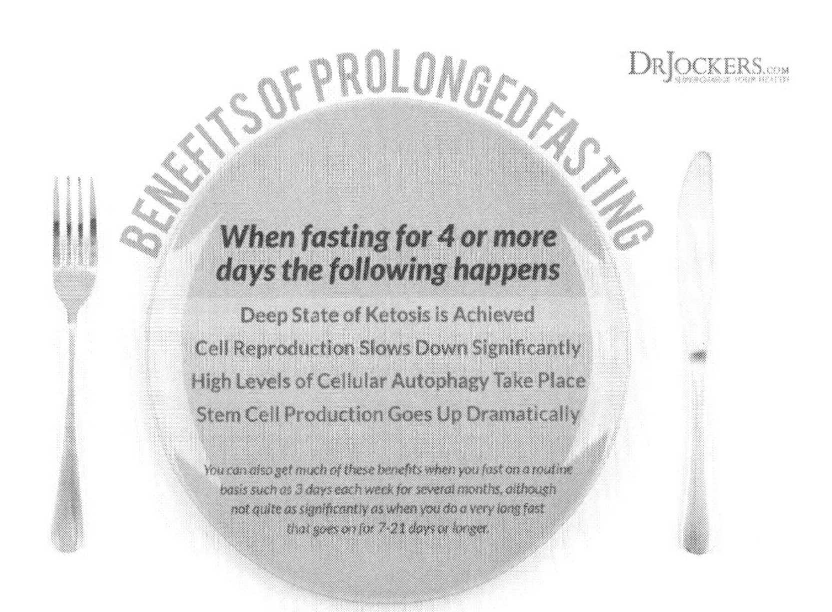

Chapter 6: Partial Fasting Strategies

Partial fasting is a way to obtain many benefits of fasting, without actually fasting. Partial fasts are low in calories and result in a significant restriction in dietary choices for a period of time. This results in a number of health improvements including a stabilized metabolism and potentially extended lifespan.

On a partial fast, you may consume up to 40% of your normal caloric total. For the average person, the daily caloric intake is about 2000 calories. This would mean the average person would follow a partial fasting protocol with a **maximum** of 800 calories per day. By dropping calories even lower to 500, typically more fasting-like benefits will be seen.

Partial fasting is a great option when:

- You are new to fasting and would like to start adapting your body
- Your body has not responded well to water fasting in the past
- You would like the benefits of fasting without losing weight

There are 5 partial fasting strategies we will discuss in this Chapter:

1. Bone Broth Fasting
2. Green Juice Fasting
3. Fasting Mimicking Diet® (FMD®)
4. Fat Fasting or Keto Fasting
5. The Daniel Fast

Included in this chapter is the Fasting Mimicking Diet® (FMD®) created by Dr. Valter Longo, PhD. Dr. Longo's approach is slightly different when it comes to caloric needs. The FMD Is 5 days long where Day 1 allows for 1100 calories and days 2–5 allow for 800.

Generally speaking, there are two styles of partial fasting strategies. One restricts all food categories but one. For example, if someone chose to eat only potatoes for several days and cut out every other food – one might call this a potato fast (apparently people actually do this). As we will talk about shortly, bone broth, green juice, and fat fasting are options in this category that are effective.

The other style of partial fast is one that may exclude some foods but derives most of its benefits from short-term yet significant caloric restriction. In this style, you may be able to eat a relatively normal whole-foods diet as long as you only consume 40% or less of your normal caloric needs. The options we will discuss in this category are the Fasting Mimicking Diet® (FMD®) and the Daniel Fast.

Bone Broth Fasting

Bone broth is a traditional and nourishing food with an important role in human nutrition dating back thousands of years. After hunting an animal, our early ancestors would feast on the organs, then the meat, and finally they would steep the bones in boiling water to extract every bit of nutrition they could get.

Bone broth is a super food containing, well, all the things you need for healthy bones and connective tissues including:

- **Collagen** – the most abundant protein in the body which maintains the structure of our bones, skin, blood vessels, and organs
- **Glucosamine & Chondroitin** – which promote healthy joints and cartilage
- **Hyaluronic Acid** – an important compound for hydrating joints and skin
- **Amino Acids** – particularly proline, glycine, and glutamine which are often lacking in meat-heavy diets
- **Minerals** like potassium, selenium, calcium, magnesium, sulfur, phosphorus, and silicon

Bone broth is very easy to digest, great for a damaged gut, and full of nutrition. This makes it excellent combined with fasting.

A bone broth fast is when you abstain from all solid foods and instead consume bone broth and water only for a period of time. While you will not be in a truly fasted state, there are still several benefits to be had from cutting out solid foods and loading up on nutritious bone broth, including:

Healing a Damaged Gut and Reducing Food Sensitivities

The highly processed westernized diets that many of us were raised on wreak havoc on our digestive systems. The high amount of sugar, processed foods, genetically-modified foods, antibiotics, alcohol, preservatives, grains, and more can cause long-term problems with digestion and overall health

You may have heard the term "leaky gut" to describe a condition in which undigested food particles leak through the intestine and into the bloodstream, often causing inflammation, food sensitivities, and ultimately autoimmune diseases (1).

Bone broth is rich in all the things that support a healthy gut like collagen, glutamine, and glycine. Fasting on bone broth can give the gut a rest and provide healing nutrients, accelerating gut healing rapidly.

Accelerating the Repair of Joints, Tendons, and Ligaments

Bone broth is the perfect solution of compounds for healthy joints and connective tissues. Collagen is gel-like and provides lubrication for joints. Collagen also makes up the structure of ligaments and tendons which are responsible for holding muscles and bones together.

Glucosamine and chondroitin provide structure for cartilage, which cushions joints, while hyaluronic acid provides lubrication.

Many people have seen great improvements in joint pain through bone broth fasting.

Reducing Signs of Aging by Improving Hair and Skin Health

70% of the protein in your skin is collagen. Studies have shown that consuming collagen can reduce the appearance of stretch marks, cellulite, and even make skin more moisturized (2, 3).

Collagen also gives hair a healthy structure.

Fasting on bone broth is a great way to replenish collagen stores rapidly and provide your body with the building blocks to keep skin and hair healthy.

Supporting a Healthy Weight Loss Plan

While bone broth is rich in nutrients and protein, it is relatively low in calories. Naturally, a bone broth fast would assist in weight loss due to caloric restriction. Many people find that bone broth is very satiating, making it quite easy to abstain from other foods.

The lack of calories will also lower insulin levels and promote fat burning.

Additionally, providing the body with glycine, arginine, and glutamine help to support the metabolism and promote lean muscle health.

Improving the Immune System and Detoxification

Part of having a healthy functioning immune system is having optimized detoxification in the liver.

Sulfur, selenium, and glycine found in bone broth support Phase II liver detoxification. Additionally, glycine assists in the production of glutathione, the body's master regulator of detoxification.

Tips for Completing a Bone Broth Fast

A bone broth fast is a great way to quickly heal the gut and sooth irritated joints. There are a number of factors to consider to get the most out of your bone broth fast.

1. **First, use a high-quality bone broth with:**

- A variety of pasture-raised chicken and beef bones (knuckles, chicken feet, oxtail and femur bones have high amounts of collagen) – Never use bones from conventionally raised livestock as these animals are exposed to hormones, antibiotics, pesticides, herbicides, and a variety of other toxins.

- Use a dash of vinegar to raise the acidity and draw the minerals out of the bones
- Simmer for at least 10-hours
- Add organic vegetables for flavor like celery, onions, and garlic
- Use anti-inflammatory components like turmeric and ginger root

**Note: You can also use pre-made bone broth for this fast. The brand I trust that is widely available in the US is Kettle and Fire. The turmeric ginger, mushroom chicken, and beef broths are all incredible.

2. **Aim to drink 24–48 oz. each day of the fast.**
3. **Choose a time frame that is challenging but not overwhelming. Common bone broth fasting windows range from 3–7 days.**
4. **Store and drink bone broth in glass containers. Plastics can leach estrogen-mimicking chemicals that are disruptive to your hormones, especially when exposed to warm liquids.**
5. **Ensure you are also drinking plenty of filtered water (Around 64 oz. per day)**
6. **Maintain light exercise during the fasting period. Taking regular walks is a great idea.**
7. **Set aside extra time to rest or nap as your energy levels may fluctuate.**

A Note on Histamine Intolerance

Bone broth is relatively high in histamines and free glutamates. While most people can metabolize these compounds just fine, those with histamine intolerance can experience headaches, trouble sleeping, dizziness, rapid heartbeat, anxiety, nasal congestion, and other symptoms associated with allergies.

If you are someone who has histamine intolerance, bone broth fasting may not be a good strategy for you.

Green Juice Fasting

Green juice fasting is when you abstain from solid food and only consume juiced greens along with water.

Greens are dense sources of vitamins, minerals, enzymes, chlorophyll, and powerful polyphenols. They are also very low in calories. The problem is that most greens are difficult to eat in mass quantities as they can be quite difficult to digest.

Juicing allows massive amounts of greens to be condensed into a single glass, providing dense nutrition without all of the digestion. Fasting with green juices boosts the healing effect and provides a long list of benefits:

Heals the Gut and Improves Digestion

The combination of fasting, dense micronutrients, and enzymes creates a great anti-inflammatory environment for the digestive tract. Including bitter greens like cilantro can help with bile flow in the liver which has many benefits including better digestion and elimination.

Strengthens the Immune System

A large portion of your immune system resides within your gut. When digestion gets backed up or there are unwanted bugs in the intestines, this puts a lot of stress on the body. Green juice fasting allows the digestive tract to clear out while providing a huge immunity boost.

Improves Cellular Oxygen Levels

A number of things like poor breathing patterns, EMFs, sedentary lifestyles, infections, and pollution can lower cellular oxygenation. Chlorophyll-rich vegetables can increase cellular oxygenation by acting similar to hemoglobin and assisting in the transport of oxygen. Chlorophyll has been shown to provide wound-healing, anti-cancer, and DNA protective effects (4).

Improves Skin Health

Through the combination of healing the gut, improving liver function, and hydrating the body; most people experience a significant improvement in their skin health.

Speeds Detoxification

Our bodies are constantly exposed to toxic compounds. We have a number of built-in systems to deal with these toxins, however, we have a much greater exposure to toxins now than ever before. This makes diligent detoxification support incredibly important.

There are external toxins like pesticides in food, chemicals in personal care products, heavy metals, mold, prescription drugs, flame retardants in furniture or paint, and a lot more.

Internal toxins could be things like byproducts of gut bacteria, byproducts of chronic inflammation, excess hormones (like estrogen), and yeast.

While it is impossible to avoid these things, green juice fasting can speed detoxification by binding to toxins in the blood, promoting liver function, healing the digestive tract, and supporting the kidneys.

Promotes Weight Loss

Fasting naturally leads to weight loss so there is no surprise here. Green juice assists with fasting in that it helps the body get rid of toxins, helps balance nutritional deficiencies, and reduces cravings.

Greens also supply a significant amount of magnesium which helps balance blood sugar and improve energy levels.

Increases Alkalinity

Human blood is designed to remain slightly alkaline at a pH of 7.365. While this pH never changes, the body can edge toward acidic or alkaline state that the body has to compensate for by leeching minerals from the bones or through other means.

Maintaining a proper pH balance is critical for optimal health. With chronic stress along with the high consumption of processed foods, added sugars, and grains; many people err to the side of acidic.

Green juices are alkaline and can assist with balancing the body's pH.

Improves Mental Function

There are over 200 chemicals that can damage and disrupt brain function (5). Common symptoms of neurotoxicity include memory loss, inability to focus, fatigue, depression, and in bad cases, seizures.

Greens have been shown to help with the elimination of certain toxins by binding them in the blood and assisting with liver function.

Building Your Green Juice

When you are constructing your green juices, you want to maximize the benefits while ensuring you stay as close to zero calories as possible. In order to do this, try choosing one green from each of the categories below.

1. **Hydrating Greens: Cucumbers, Celery, Bok Choy**

   Cucumbers are full of water and silica. Silica is important for connective tissue health. This includes bones, joints, skin, hair, and nails. They are also a good source of potassium, magnesium, and vitamin C.

   Celery is also rich in water, silica, and electrolytes.

Bok Choy contains over 70 antioxidants and is full of electrolytes.

2. **Chlorophyll-Rich Greens: Spinach, Arugula, Kale, Collard Greens, Watercress, Spirulina, and Chlorella**

As we discussed already, chlorophyll is healthy for many reasons. Dark leafy greens as well as Spirulina and chlorella are excellent sources of chlorophyll.

Dark leafy greens are also a great source of Vitamin A, Vitamin E, and Vitamin K.

Kale is rich in sulforaphane which raises glutathione in the body and helps to neutralize toxins.

Spirulina and Chlorella are power foods that are loaded with chlorophyll, contain essential amino acids, and help to purify the blood.

Researched benefits of chlorella include cholesterol improvements, improvement in blood sugar balance, anti-inflammation, anti-cancer, and protection from heart disease (6).

Spirulina has many of the same benefits (7).

3. **Anti-Inflammatory Herbs and Roots: Cilantro, Mint, Parsley, Ginger, Turmeric**

Bitter herbs assist with bile flow from the liver which assists in the expulsion of toxins through the colon. This also assists with digestion. Bitter herbs like cilantro are also known as being weak chelators of heavy metals in the body which can help rid them form the body.

Ginger helps to reduce inflammation in the intestines, reduce gas, assist with bowel movements, increase bile flow.

Turmeric is great for reducing inflammation throughout the body, detoxifying the liver, and raising glutathione levels. Turmeric is one of the most studied foods ever and may help with a wide array of conditions including arthritis, heart disease, digestive disorders, diabetes, depression, fibromyalgia, and cancer.

4. **Acidic Fruits: Lemons, Limes, Green Apples**

   Lemons and Limes are rich in Vitamin C and bioflavonoids. Vitamin C is an essential antioxidant and has the added benefit of protecting the nutrients in your juice from oxidation. This means more nutrition for you.

   Green apples contain acetic acid that help combat bad bugs in the gut. It also improves liver and gallbladder function.

Tips for Green Juice Fasting

1. Always use organic ingredients. Not doing this could mean you are mainlining pesticides, herbicides, and heavy metals into your body instead of all the good stuff.
2. Buy local and fresh produce whenever possible.
3. If you buy store-bought juices, make sure they have not been pasteurized and do not contain any sugar.
4. Drink your juices immediately, many of the nutrients will become oxidized with time and become less beneficial
5. Again, it is best to store and consume liquids from glass instead of plastic due to estrogen mimicking compounds.

Fasting Mimicking Diet

The Fasting Mimicking Diet®, or FMD®, is a high-nutrition, low-protein, low-carbohydrate meal plan in which calories are restricted for five days out of a month.

Developed by Valter Longo, PhD, a professor of gerontology and biological sciences at the University of Southern California and the head of the Longevity Institute - The FMD is designed to generate similar benefits to fasting, but without the complete restriction of calories.

After being granted a patent for the FMD protocol, Dr. Longo released his program called the ProLon® five-day FMD. His goal was to minimize hunger while deriving as many fasting benefits as possible.

Several studies have been conducted on Fasting Mimicking Diets and show that they are capable of:

Promoting Healthy Aging

Studies have shown that fasting mimicking diets reduces risk factors for aging and all-cause mortality (8). This is likely primarily through improvements in blood sugar, cholesterol, and inflammation.

Promoting Healthy Weight Loss

Fasting mimicking diets shifts the body into a state of ketosis which allows the body to burn stored fat more easily.

Following a 5-day FMD cycle for 3 months in a row was shown to reduce body fat and overall body weight.

Lowering Blood Sugar and Insulin

By putting your body in a hypo-caloric state for 5-days, you give your pancreas and insulin receptors adequate time to reset themselves.

The FMD was found specifically to help reverse late stage Type 2 as well as some cases of Type 1 diabetes.

Decreasing Blood Pressure

By reestablishing blood sugar and insulin levels that are healthy, the body can regulate electrolytes and hydration levels more effectively. This tends to result in a return to normal blood pressure.

Improving Cholesterol

Following an FMD has been shown to reduce total and LDL cholesterol while also increasing HDL (9). This allows for better LDL to HDL ratios and ultimately more favorable triglyceride levels.

Reducing Autoimmunity

In a mouse model, the FMD was shown to reduce the severity of multiple sclerosis while completely reversing symptoms in 20% (10). The authors concluded that this was through a mediation of autoimmunity within the body.

Assisting in Healing Inflammatory Bowel Disease

Fasting mimicking diets may assist with healing from IBD by reducing intestinal inflammation, increasing stem cells within the gut, and promoting the growth of beneficial gut bacteria (11).

Protecting Brain Function

One of the hallmarks of dementia and neurodegenerative disorders is the slowing down of neurogenesis. Neurogenesis is the process in which new neurons are formed in the brain. Evidence suggests that following an FMD may promote neurogenesis in the hippocampus and provide protective effects against Alzheimer's and other types of dementia (12).

Fasting mimicking diets have been studied in both animal and human models. These studies support the dietary approach as being very safe with no major side effects (13).

Implementing A Fasting Mimicking Diet

While you can simply purchase Dr. Longo's FMD package with the food already included, you can also follow the guidelines below to design your own.

Preparing for a 5-day FMD (5–7 Days Leading Up to an FMD)

- Consume a low-protein diet (0.36 grams of protein per pound of bodyweight per day)
  - Ex: 160 lb. individual would consume only 57.6 grams of protein in a day
- Consume mostly vegetables and fish
- Consider taking a multivitamin and an Omega-3 supplement

FMD Protocol

Day 1 – Priming the body for a transition into fasting

Total Calories: 1,100

500 calories from complex carbs, 500 from healthy fats, and 25 grams of plant-based protein.

Recommended protein source: nuts

Days 2-5 – Shifting into ketosis, accelerating autophagy, and promoting stem cell regeneration

Total Calories: 800

400 calories from complex carbs, 400 from healthy fats

Day 6 (Transition Day):

This is the transition back into a normal diet. It is recommended that calories on transition day should come mostly from complex carbohydrates like vegetables, wild rice, fruit, legumes, etc. It is recommended to avoid high amounts of meats, saturated fats, and dairy.

Additional Guidelines for a Fasting Mimicking Diet are as Follows:

- Low protein and low carbohydrates
- No or minimal animal products
- Preferred healthy fats are nuts, avocado, olives and olive oil
- Complex carbs include most vegetables
- Up to 4 cups of sugarless tea are allowed
- No water restrictions (drink as much as you want)
- Coffee not recommended
- A multivitamin and an Omega-3 supplement are recommended

How Often to Do a Fasting Mimicking Diet

Based on the recommendations provided by Valter Longo and the Prolon team, how often you perform an FMD depends on your current health issues and goals. These recommendations are below.

Once a Month for someone who:

- Has **2 risk factors** for diabetes, cancer, cardiovascular disease, or neurodegenerative disease AND is **obese** or **overweight**

Once Every Two Months for someone who:

- Has **2 risk factors** for diabetes, cancer, cardiovascular disease, or neurodegenerative disease and are **average weight**

Once Every Three Months for someone who:

- Has **1 risk factor** for diabetes, cancer, cardiovascular disease, or neurodegenerative disease and is **average weight**

Once Every Four Months for someone who:

- Is **healthy**, follows a normal diet, and **is not physically active**

Once Every Six Months for someone who:

- Is **healthy**, follows a healthy diet, and **is physically active**

****NOTE: My recommendations on fasting frequency differ slightly and I will be covering them in Chapter 8: How to Begin Fasting**

Fat or Keto Fast

Fat fasting is a great way to accelerate weight loss on a ketogenic diet or simply provide a more comfortable mode of approaching a fast.

Fat fasting is essentially eating nothing but healthy fats in moderate amounts. This helps provide satiating fuel for the body while supporting a state of ketosis. Pushing the body into a state of ketosis in itself is a fasting-mimicking diet that provides many of the same benefits as fasting.

As we covered in detail in the beginning of this book, shifting into a state of ketosis has several benefits including: lowering inflammation, improving metabolic disorders, protecting against neurodegenerative disease, calming anxiety, improving depression, protecting against cancer, and improving mitochondrial health.

A fat fast can be done as part of an intermittent fasting routine as well as an extended fast.

When You Might Want to Consider a Fat Fast:

- **As an introduction to a Ketogenic Diet** – This can help rapidly shift the body into ketosis while remaining satiated.
- **Intermittent Fasting** Aid – Have a butter coffee for breakfast to satiate and place your body in ketosis. This can help maintain longer daily fasts.
- **If Your Body Has Not Responded Well to Water Fasting** – Many people find when they don't respond well to water fasting that fat fasting is much more doable.

How to Implement a Fat Fast

- Design a high-fat, low-calorie meal plan. You want to consume somewhere between 500 to 1000 calories at most per day. 90% or more of your calories should come from fats.
- Aim to follow this plan for 2–7 days.
- Consume healthy fats such as avocado, coconut oil, olive oil, grass-fed butter, MCT Oil, and pastured eggs.
- Other acceptable foods include leafy greens, non-starchy vegetables, herbs, coffee, lemons, and limes.
- Exogenous Ketones may be taken during a fat fast to assist the shift into ketosis and stave off hunger.

Example of an Intermittent Fat Fast Meal Plan

Morning:

Coffee with 1 tbsp. of grass-fed butter, 1 tsp of MCT oil, and 1 tbsp. of whipping cream.

Mid-day:

Consume regular meal or fast until dinner.

Dinner:

Consume a regular meal

Example of Extended Fat Fast Daily Meal Plan

Morning:

Coffee with 1 tbsp. of grass-fed butter, 1 tsp of MCT oil, and 1 tbsp. of whipping cream.

Mid-Day:

1–2 Cups of Leafy Greens with 1 Avocado with 2 tbsp. of olive oil, 1 tbsp. of lemon juice and herb dressing

Remainder of the Day:

Fast. Only drink water or herbal tea. Salt, electrolytes, and exogenous ketones can be used to reduce hunger and improve energy levels.

Do this for 2–7 days.

Following this plan for 3–7 days will achieve many of the benefits of fasting including burning fat, raising ketone levels, increasing HGH, promoting autophagy, and stimulating stem cell development.

Daniel Fast

The Daniel fast is a spiritual fasting strategy based on the biblical account of a prophet named Daniel.

Detailed in two chapters of the Bible, Daniel fasted from meat, wine, and stimulating foods while focusing on praying and seeking god. Many Christians have followed the Daniel fast in order to heal the body while seeking a deeper connection to God.

The Daniel Fast includes vegetables, fruits, legumes, nuts, seeds, grains, healthy fats, and water. While this is not really a fast, it is a partial fast temporarily cutting out meat, dairy, sugar, and processed foods.

While some people report receiving health benefits during the Daniel fast, the true purpose is to limit your stimulation from food so that one can focus fully on having a deep connection with God.

The Daniel fast is typically followed for 10–21 days. Being a plant-based vegan diet, you would run the risk of experiencing nutrient deficiencies if followed for too long. For this reason, I would not recommend following a Daniel fast for longer than 21 days.

The Story of Daniel

In the Old Testament, the book of Daniel describes Daniels fast for two chapters.

In Daniel 1:12–20, King Nebuchadnezzar attempted to convince Daniel and his friends to consume the royal foods (including meats, breads and other dense foods) so that they can be "strong and healthy".

Daniel believed the kings foods to be unhealthy and instead proposed an experiment.

He would consume only vegetables and water for 10 days and then compare his health to the men eating the royal food.

After doing so, Daniel and his friends appeared to be healthier and stronger. It was written that this fast from rich foods provided Daniel with heightened wisdom, spiritual understanding, and health.

Daniel later proceeded to fast for three weeks and again achieved answered prayer and deep spiritual insight.

How to Follow a Modernized Daniel Fast

Foods to Include – Foods grown from seeds: vegetables, fruits, whole grains, nuts, seeds, legumes, and healthy fats.

Vegetables

Organic, Fresh or Frozen: artichokes, asparagus, beets, broccoli, Brussels sprouts, cabbage, carrots, cauliflower, celery, chili peppers, collard greens, cucumbers, eggplant, garlic, ginger root, kale, leeks, lettuce, mushrooms, mustard greens, okra, onions, parsley, potatoes, radishes, rutabagas, scallions, spinach, sprouts, squashes, sweet potatoes, tomatoes, turnips, watercress, yams, and zucchini.

Fruits

Organic, Fresh or Frozen low-glycemic: lemons, limes, berries, granny smith apples, and grapefruit (Limited to ½ cup each of berries, apples, and grapefruit per day)

Higher Glycemic fruits: apricots, oranges, apples, bananas, cantaloupe, cherries, figs, grapes, guava, honeydew, kiwi, mangoes, nectarines, papayas, peaches, pears, pineapple, watermelon (limited to ¼ cup per day)

Healthy Fats

Avocados, avocado oil, olives, extra virgin olive oil, coconut, coconut butter, and coconut oil.

Whole Grains

While whole grains are typically included in a Daniel fast, I recommend limiting these to only one cup of sprouted grain per day. Consuming too many grains can cause blood sugar issues and digestive disturbances.

Grain options include gluten-free oats, brown rice, quinoa, and buckwheat.

Beans and Legumes

These are high in starch and carbohydrates. They are also irritating to the digestive tract. Similar to grains, beans and legumes should be limited to ½ cup daily.

It is best to buy these organic, soak them overnight, and cook them thoroughly. Pressure cooking can make these more digestible as well.

Beans and legumes to include in a Daniel fast include pinto beans, black beans, kidney beans, cannellini beans, white beans, split peas, black-eyed peas, and lentils.

Nuts and Seeds

Nuts and seeds are good sources of protein and healthy fats. Many people have trouble digesting them, however.

Choose raw, sprouted, or dry roasted nuts with no added oils. Including, but not limited to, almonds, brazil nuts, hazelnuts, pecans, cashews, macadamia nuts, and walnuts.

Seeds like flax, chia, pumpkin, sunflower, and hemp are all great options as well.

You can also include nut butters that do not have added sugar, preservatives, or vegetable oils.

Herbs and Spices

Season your foods well with organic fresh or dried herbs including turmeric, ginger, thyme, basil, oregano, sage, cilantro, oregano, rosemary, star anise, cumin, coriander, cardamom, cinnamon, and any other herb or spice that does not contain sugar or msg.

Beverages

Filtered water is mostly what you should be drinking.

Other acceptable beverages are nut milks, green juices, and herbal teas with no added sugar or preservatives.

Coffee is not recommended. If you are an avid coffee drinker, consider limiting your intake to 1 cup in a day.

Other Optional Foods

Plant-based protein powder

Fermented Vegetables

Apple Cider Vinegar

Small amounts of stevia or monk fruit

Foods to Exclude on a Daniel Fast

- All Meat and Dairy
- All sugars and sweeteners (this includes natural sweeteners like honey and maple syrup)
- All leavened bread and baked goods
- All refined and processed foods
- Highly processed oils (margarine, canola oil, corn oil, vegetable oil, soybean oil, sunflower oil, grapeseed oil, safflower oil, rice bran oil, peanut oil, sesame oil)
- Fast Foods
- Beverages other than those listed above

Tips for Success on a Daniel Fast

- Begin cutting out processed foods one week before starting – this is a good time to taper caffeine and sugar off
- Clear your schedule during the fasting period so you can focus on what is important to you
- Drink at least 64oz of water each day
- Set aside time for daily study, prayer, worship, and journaling
- Partake in gentle daily exercise like walking in nature
- Get consistent sleep
- Add a bit of salt to your water for electrolytes
- Consider hiring a health coach or an accountability partner to keep you on track
- Consider implementing a daily intermittent fasting schedule along with the Daniel fast for improved benefits and heightened mental clarity

Advantages of Partial Fasting Compared to Water Fasting

Easier and Generally Safer

While water fasting isn't particularly dangerous for most people, it still has its risks. It is also only recommended that you complete an extended water fast after you've become very comfortable with 24-hour fasts and daily intermittent fasting. Partial fasting is much more tolerable for people new to fasting or who have not responded well to water fasting in the past.

More Doable for People Taking Medication

Many medications can be hard on the digestive tract when taken without food on a regular basis. The same goes with supplements. In fact, some supplements don't get absorbed very well without some dietary fat present.

If you are taking medication and/or supplements, partial fasting can be an approach that allows you to get fasting benefits and still stay on your medication regimen.

If you are considering a fast and are on medication, you should consult with a physician and have supervision to ensure there are no major adverse events.

Provides Micronutrients

The partial fasting strategies mentioned above are nutrient-dense. This allows for many of the benefits of fasting plus added nutrition that may assist in healing the body. This added nutrition may also help prevent fasting side effects like cravings, fatigue, and dizziness.

Less Weight Loss

While weight loss is a natural effect of fasting, many people are happy with their current weight and would rather maintain as much of their body mass as possible. Partaking in a partial fast is a great way to preserve muscle mass on longer fasts. Bone broth fasting is particularly helpful for this purpose.

Downsides of Partial Fasting Compared to Water Fasting

Less Autophagy

As we discussed in Chapter 2, one of the main benefits of fasting is the breaking down and recycling of old cells – called autophagy. The amount of autophagy from fasting is directly related to the intensity and duration of the fast. This means a 5-day water fast would produce significantly more autophagy than a 5-day bone broth or green juice fast.

Less Growth Hormone

Human growth hormone (HGH) tends to increase significantly during a fast. High amounts of HGH extends cell lifespan and improves cellular repair.

While intermittent and water fasting tend to create large increases in HGH, partial fasts do not create a true fasted state. This means partial fasting will not create the same surge in HGH.

Less Stem Cell Production

Fasting is particularly effective at raising stem cells within the intestines. Even a 24-hour fast can raise stem cell production within the intestines.

Since partial fasting does not actually exclude food entirely, these benefits may not be the same.

While partial fasting may not provide all of the benefits as water fasting, it is still an excellent option for those who are trying to prepare their bodies for longer fasts. Partial fasts are more tolerable and provide many fasting benefits to a lesser extent.

Chapter 7: Fasting for Chronic Disease

Several chronic diseases benefit greatly from fasting. After learning how the physiology of the body adapts to fasting, this makes perfect sense. Because fasting is able to improve the function of the body from the cellular level, it has the power to improve a wide range of diseases.

In this chapter, we are going to discuss how fasting can be applied to help in the healing process of 4 of the most common diseases of our time:

- Cancer
- Diseases of the Digestive Tract
- Autoimmunity
- Neurodegenerative Diseases

These are conditions I see often in my health coaching practice. The worst part of it all is that most doctors say there is no way to heal these things... Well, that's just simply not the case. There are many things you can do to support the body in healing.

As we cover each of these conditions, I will detail top strategies for healing in addition to fasting.

Cancer

Cancer affects around 17 million people worldwide every year. Over half of those cases end up in an early death. The four top 4 deadliest types of cancer are those of the lungs, liver, stomach, and bowels.

You may have noticed that 3 of the top 4 deadliest cancers are cancers of the digestive tract. Remember when we discussed how fasting can promote stem cell regeneration in the intestines? This might be important to consider when dealing with cancers of the digestive tract.

Some of the top risk factors for developing cancer seem to be:

- Being overweight
- Consuming a poor diet
- Having poor blood sugar control
- Being sedentary
- Certain infections
- Smoking
- Overexposure to ionizing radiation (X-rays, Certain wireless technologies)

The great news is that fasting alone can improve most of these risk factors.

Fasting Benefits and Cancer

1. **Boosts Immunity**

   The tendency that many people have to constantly eat throughout the day puts a lot of stress on the digestive system. In addition to being highly energy-intensive, poor digestion is often a source of chronic inflammation and ultimately sets the conditions for autoimmunity. Fasting gives digestion a rest while allowing the digestive tract to heal. Together this provides for a powerful reset of the immune system.

   Fasting also allows the immune system to better coordinate inflammatory cytokines Interleukin-6 and Tumor Necrosis Factor Alpha which are highly inflammatory and often elevated in those with cancer (1, 2, 3).

   There is also some evidence that fasting for longer amounts of time helps to inhibit viral and parasitic replication, which provides yet another relief to the immune system.

2. **Stimulates Autophagy**

   When autophagy is not functioning properly in the body, you get a higher instance of many diseases. In the case of cancer, cancer cells actually take control of the autophagy process and shut it off completely. This allows cancer cells to stay alive and continue to reproduce as long as the immune system does not stop them.

Physiologically speaking, cancer cells are damaged and play no beneficial role in the human body. This is exactly the type of cell that should be targeted by the immune system through autophagy.

As we've discussed several times, fasting promotes higher amounts of autophagy which helps the body get rid of cells that aren't pulling their weight. This process is especially activated at the 16–24-hour mark of a fast.

A recent review on the topic of autophagy showed that intermittent fasting is able to: (4)

- Improve the efficacy of several chemotherapy and radiation therapy-targeted cancers
- Protect healthy cells from cytotoxic therapies, while sensitizing cancer cells
- Stimulate DNA repair

The authors of this study concluded that stimulating autophagy through fasting may be one of the most cost-effective ways to regulate the survival of tumor cells.

3. Accelerates Genetic Repair

As we've discussed, fasting and caloric restriction are associated with a longer lifespan. Not only are these practices associated with a longer lifespan, but also lower instances of disease. When we look at fasting from the perspective of a cell, it seems that cells tend to live longer when there is not an excess of food around.

During fasting, cells slow down cell division. Cancer cells are literally rapidly dividing and immortal cells so this may be an important finding in the fight against cancer.

Fasting may be able to accelerate DNA repair due to its effect on growth hormone. Growth hormone surges during the night while we sleep to help repair damaged cells, promote fat burning, and retain muscle mass. When you fast, growth hormone rises significantly and stimulates these same processes.

4. **Restores Insulin Sensitivity**

Insulin surges when we eat carb-dense meals while growth hormone surges during times of fasting. This makes Insulin and growth hormone in direct competition with each other. Having high insulin levels will make it difficult to keep growth hormone levels optimized (5, 6).

The abundance of food we have in today's society, along with the high prevalence of processed and carb-dense foods, has led to an epidemic of blood sugar problems and insulin resistance. Insulin resistance sets you up for diabetes, heart disease, Alzheimer's, and cancer.

If we want to maximize the healing effect of growth hormone, then insulin must be minimized. Fasting achieves this goal very efficiently.

Specific Anti-Cancer Mechanisms That Fasting Targets

1. **Inhibiting IL-8**

Interleukin-8 (IL-8) is a proinflammatory molecule that is often elevated in tissues where tumors are present.

Elevated IL-8 levels tend to promote (7):

- Angiogenesis: the development of a blood supply for a tumor
- Metastasis: the migration of cancer cells from a tumor throughout the body
- Rapid cancer cell division

Targeting IL-8 has been a focus for some anti-cancer treatments. It has been found that fasting can effectively lower IL-8 signaling (8).

2. **Depriving Cancer Cells of Sugar**

Cancer cells are metabolically damaged, making them unable to use the same energetic processes that normal cells use.

Normal cells preferentially utilize a process called oxidative phosphorylation to create ATP from either sugar or fatty acids through a reaction with oxygen. Cancer cells, on the other hand, are unable to perform oxidative phosphorylation and undergo a fermentation reaction instead.

This fermentation primarily relies on sugar in order to work. In fact, cancer cells have an overabundance of insulin receptors – allowing them to gobble up sugar at an abnormally high rate. Luckily though, most cancer cells are unable to utilize fatty acids to generate ATP in the same way that normal cells are.

Therefore, it is generally a good idea to shift your body towards a state of ketosis in an effort to limit the ability of cancer cells to uptake sugar, create ATP, and reproduce (9).

3. **Improving White Blood Cell Function**

White blood cells are the soldiers of the immune system. Different types of white blood cells circulate throughout the body and scout for things that shouldn't be there. This includes things like bacteria, viruses, parasites, and cancer cells.

In order for white blood cells to operate well, they need an adequate supply of Vitamin C. This was discovered by Linus Pauling in the 1960's, who won a Nobel prize for his research.

In the 1970's Dr. John Ely postulated the Glucose-Ascorbate-Antagonism (GAA) Theory. What he discovered was that both glucose and Vitamin C are similar in structure and rely upon insulin in order to enter cells through the Glut-1 receptor. Another really important discovery to note is that glucose has a higher affinity for this receptor than Vitamin C.

This means that when there is elevated blood glucose, or in the case of insulin resistance, Vitamin C will not be able to absorb into cells.

Most animals are able to make their own Vitamin C endogenously. Humans do not have this capability. This means we must consume it in our diets.

Given what we know about white blood cells, Vitamin C, and sugar; naturally we would want to ensure we are consuming adequate Vitamin

C while keeping carb intake very low to optimize white blood cell function and give ourselves the best chance at fighting off cancer.

4. Up Regulating AMP-K

AMP-K stands for Adenosine Monophosphate-activated Protein Kinase. When ATP (**Adenosine Tri**phosphate) is broken down for energy within cells, phosphate groups are removed to form ADP and AMP (Adenosine **Di**phosphate and Adenosine **Mono**phosphate, respectively).

When the ratio of AMP to ATP is elevated, this signals that the body is low on energy. The AMP-K pathway is partly responsible for up regulating energy production when energy stores are low within cells.

Boosting the expression of AMP-K has been shown to:

- Divert glucose away from cancer cells and into healthy cells (10)
- Potentially reverse metabolic damage in cancer cells (11)

Fasting, restricting carbohydrates, and intense exercise have all been shown to boost AMP-K expression (12, 13).

5. Inhibiting mTOR

mTOR stands for mammalian target of rapamycin. The mTOR pathway plays a role in regulating cell growth and division. For example, when you exercise a muscle to make it stronger, mTOR will up regulate after your workout to build more muscle in the areas you worked out.

We know that tissues with cancer present have an elevated expression of mTOR signaling which is thought to play a role in the rapid growth of tumors.

While some expression of mTOR is needed to stay healthy, an over expression can contribute to cancer growth. Consequently, insulin is one of the primary activators of mTOR.

Other activators of mTOR include:

- Proteins with a high amount of leucine
- Excessive calories

- High carb intake
- Exercise

Naturally, fasting and ketogenic dieting are able to drastically lower mTOR and potentially slow the growth of many types of cancer (14, 15).

Ideally you want temporary surges in mTOR with prolonged bouts of mTOR inhibition between. This make intermittent fasting with ketogenic nutrition a powerful strategy against cancer.

6. Stimulating Apoptosis of Defective Cells

Naturally, when cells in the body become old or damaged, they self-destruct to make room for new healthy cells. This process is called apoptosis and is mostly absent in cancer cells.

In order for cancer cells to remain alive and healthy, they must have a strong supply of glucose. As we just discussed, cancer cells rely almost entirely on glucose for energy.

In a recent study, authors noted that short-term fasting from 24–72 hours was able to stimulate cancer cell death (apoptosis) by shifting cellular metabolism from glycolysis (the cancer cells preferred state) to oxidative phosphorylation and the metabolism of fatty acids for energy. Because cancer cells have a very weak ability to metabolize through oxidative phosphorylation, they quickly die (16).

The authors of this study postulate that fasting not only promotes apoptosis, but also heightens cancer cells' vulnerability to therapies such as chemotherapy.

It is critical to maintain a strict nutrition protocol such a ketogenic meal plan when not fasting to prevent a rebound effect that could actually promote cancer growth.

Prolonged Fasting for Cancer

During a fast, healthy cells become highly resilient to stress. At the same time, cancer cells seem to become vulnerable to apoptosis either by the immune system or external therapies like chemotherapy and radiation.

Longer fasts may be an effective tool to create an environment within your body that cancer cells do not survive well in. Longer fasts are advantageous over shorter fasts in this case in that they restrict glucose to the cell significantly, promote a state of ketosis, and create substantial amounts of autophagy.

While intermittent fasting can be great for metabolic conditions, my experience has shown me that prolonged fasting can be a powerful tool in cancer healing.

A strategy that I have seen success with is performing a 48–72 fast, once per week to gain the benefits we discussed above and provide time each week for your body to target the cancer cells within your body.

I have had particular clients partake in a 21-day fast for advanced healing. This is not for everyone and should be monitored very closely by a health care practitioner.

Plant-based Ketogenic Nutrition

What you eat outside of your fasting windows is just as important as the fasting windows themselves. As I briefly mentioned in the previous sections of this chapter, improper re-feeding between fasts can accelerate cancer growth if done improperly.

One of the key components of fasting for cancer healing is restricting glucose from cancer cells. This is why I recommend combining fasting with a plant-based ketogenic diet.

This ensures that, even upon re-feeding, you continue to support a state of ketosis while also providing dense nutrition to support the immune system. This puts cancer cells at a large metabolic disadvantage and makes them less likely to survive.

In addition to staying in ketosis, a plant-based ketogenic diet is lower in protein which helps to limit activation of the mTOR pathway within the body. As we discussed previously, mTOR is highly involved with rapid tissue growth and tends to be overly expressed in cancerous lesions. In addition to insulin, protein is a major activator of mTOR expression.

Finally, filling the diet with certain types of plant foods provides nutrients that have been found to inhibit cancer growth. These include things like EGCG in green tea, sulforaphane in broccoli sprouts, curcumin from turmeric, and anthocyanin in dark berries.
For a more in-depth explanation of this, I have an extensive article on drjockers.com that details how to follow a plant-based ketogenic diet for cancer. Just search Plant-based Keto on my website and you will find it.

I also have an online program called the Cancer Cleanse Program that provides a meal plan, shopping guides, video guides, and advanced healing techniques to maximize your body's natural healing defenses.

Fasting Mimicking Diet

One of the common major side effects with chemotherapy and radiation is rapid weight loss. If someone is already very thin and undergoing cancer treatment, fasting may not be the best option.

To obtain many of the same benefits without promoting further weight loss, an FMD may be the best option.

Hyperbaric Oxygen Therapy (HBOT)

We discussed briefly that cancer cells use a metabolic process called glycolysis to produce energy. Glycolysis is anaerobic, meaning that it occurs in the absence of oxygen. This is the opposite of normal healthy cells, which prefer a rich supply of oxygen to produce energy efficiently.

This means that enriching the bloodstream with oxygen may be a beneficial strategy for boosting the health of normal cells while fighting cancer cells.

A 2020 study conducted on 24 patients diagnosed with late-stage metastatic gastric cancer found that combining chemotherapy, fasting, ketogenic diet, hyperthermia (warming of the tissue), and HBOT had a significant impact in 22 out of the 24 patients (17).

Another similar study, also published in 2020, observed patients with late-stage metastatic pancreatic cancer. Again, when chemotherapy was administered with a ketogenic diet, hyperthermia, and HBOT – survival outcomes were increased (18).

Another study found similar results with metastatic lung cancer patients (19).

There numerous other case studies which used similar approaches and found drastic improvements in late-stage cancer patients.

In fact, a lot of research is being directed towards these types of approaches for cancer. In fact, Dr. Thomas Seyfried, who is considered one of the leading researchers on the metabolic defects of cancer cells, proposed something called the Press-pulse method for cancer treatment (20).

In this method, Seyfried suggests creating cycles of stress on cancer cells by utilizing specifically timed bouts of fasting, ketogenic diet, hyperbaric oxygen therapy, radiation, and chemotherapy.

Daily Detoxification

It is impossible to avoid everything that is bad for the body. We all encounter toxins whether they are from polluted air, electronics, paint in our homes, or an endless number of other sources. Toxins are a stressor that we cannot avoid.

What we can do is support our bodies ability to get rid of these things so that it can expend energy on other important processes.

Fasting is one strategy that accelerates the elimination of toxins. In addition to this you will also want to:

- Hydrate very well
- Use herbs that support detoxification pathways
- Sweat through exercise and/or sauna use
- Consider using coffee enemas to clear the colon, stimulate the liver, and raise glutathione levels

There are many ways you can support detoxification that I cover in depth on my website. These are also things I cover in my Cancer Cleanse program.

Conventional Cancer Therapies

As we have discussed, fasting tends to improve the efficacy of chemotherapy and radiation (21). This may be because fasting restricts fuel supply to cancer cells and sensitizes them to other stressors.

A 2009 case study report documented the experience of 10 patients who were undergoing high-dose chemotherapy and elected to undergo various fasting protocols (22). The fasting ranges for these patients ranged from 48–140 hours leading up to their chemotherapy treatments as well as 5–56 hours following treatment.

The authors of this report observed that these 10 patients were able to avoid common side effects of chemotherapy such as fatigue, weakness, and digestive upset by fasting leading up to and following treatment.

The best part about this is that these patients avoided side effects without lessening the effectiveness of the chemotherapy.

Another 2016 study separated 20 patients into 3 groups: (23)

- 24-hour fast leading up to platinum-based chemotherapy
- 48-hour fast leading up to platinum-based chemotherapy
- 72-hour fast (48 hours leading up to and 24 hours following platinum-based chemotherapy)

The authors of this study found that longer fasting windows were associated with lower inflammation markers and DNA damage indicators following treatment. All fasting groups experienced a lower instance of chemotherapy side-effects.

Finally, a 2018 study implemented a 60-hour fasting protocol split into a 36 hour fast before treatment and 24 hours following (24).

The authors of this study concluded that fasting improved quality of life during chemotherapy treatment by reducing side effects such as fatigue.

A suggested protocol based on the Press-pulse method proposed by Dr. Seyfried is to:

1. Follow a ketogenic meal plan
2. Fast at least 14-hours leading up to a chemotherapy or radiation treatment
3. Break the fast shortly after treatment
4. Consume plenty of plant-based anti-cancer foods and receive HBOT in the following days
5. Follow up with subsequent fasting cycles and ketogenic eating

Another expert in the field of natural cancer treatment, Dr. Nasha Winters, has some great protocols. Here are some ideas based on her work:

- Following a 13-hour fast on a daily basis (this alone lowers cancer recurrence by an amazing 70%)
- Implementing 2, 16–18-hour fasts on 2 non-consecutive days out of the week.
- Implementing a 3-day fast, once per month
- Fasting for 3 days (72 hours), leading up to chemotherapy and radiation treatment
- **For very thin patients,** following a Fasting Mimicking Diet can be great around cancer treatments to prevent cachexia while lowering the side effects of cancer treatment
- **Very thin patients** can also benefit from supplementing with essential amino acids or partaking in bone broth fasting around times of treatment

Dr. Nasha has a great book called The Metabolic Approach to Cancer that dives into these strategies and is an excellent resource for taking control of the body's ability to fight cancer.

Digestive Health

According to the National Institute of Diabetes and Digestive and Kidney Diseases, 60–70 million people are affected by some kind of digestive disease in the US each year (25). Out of those, almost 50 million require a doctor's treatment or a visit to the emergency room.

Some of the most common digestive diseases include:

- Chronic Constipation

- Diverticulosis/Diverticulitis
- Gallstones
- Acid Reflux
- Irritable Bowel Syndrome
- Ulcerative Colitis
- Liver Disease
- Peptic Ulcers

Through a wide array of different beneficial effects, fasting is able to improve many of these conditions and make them less likely to occur in the first place.

Fasting Benefits for Digestive Health

There is no single specific thing about fasting that makes it beneficial for so many diseases. It is instead, the huge number of small improvements within human physiology that occur when fasting that allow the body to become more efficient and heal.

One major way in which fasting has such a major impact on health is the healing of the digestive tract.

The digestive tract is very fragile. The intestinal lining is just one layer of cells thick, and this layer is a primary key of our immune system! If this lining becomes compromised, not only might you have digestive issues, but also immune issues, neurological issues, and chronic inflammation throughout the body.

Here are some of the ways fasting helps improve digestive health.

1. **Intestinal Stem Cell Regeneration**

   Every cell in your body has a renewal rate. Some tissues replace their cells much more quickly than others. While some organs will grow 100% new cells within days or weeks, other tissues take several months or even years to do the same.

   The intestinal tract has one of the highest cell turnover rates. With age, cell turnover slows down throughout the body due to lower stem cell counts.

Several studies have observed that fasting can enhance stem cell function in the digestive tract (26).

A study performed in mice found that a 24-hour fast was able to produce this effect in both young and old mice (27).

The implications of up regulated stem cell production may be that fasting can accelerate the healing of intestinal damage, help to restore the gut barrier, and completely reverse the chronic inflammation cascade that occurs after that barrier is breached.

2. **Reduces Inflammation**

Inflammation is a double-edged sword. When in appropriate amounts, it guides the immune system to heal. In excess amounts, it can cause diseases of many different types.

Since your gut is one of the ultimate barriers to every other inner working of your body, chronic inflammation here is not good. Common digestive diseases related to chronic inflammation include irritable bowel disease (IBD) and ulcerative colitis.

Fasting quickly mitigates this inflammation fortunately.

A study done on Ramadan fasting found that sixty patients with ulcerative colitis experienced reduced symptoms after Ramadan (28).

Additionally, a Fasting Mimicking Diet has been shown to provide similar benefits. One study conducted by Dr. Valter Longo found that after 4 days on an FMD, there was a significant reduction of intestinal inflammation, increased stem cells, and promoted gut-protective bacteria (29). Water fasting was used as a comparative therapy in this study and was found to provide similar benefits.

3. **Restoring the Gut Barrier**

This benefit should be very apparent by now, but I want to touch on it one more time. The gut barrier is one of your strongest defenses against foreign invaders within the body. When the gut lining is compromised, you get chronic inflammation, poor digestion, and all kinds of autoimmune diseases. Having a leaky gut also predisposes you to heart disease and mood disorders.

Considering that fasting lowers inflammation and increases stem cell production in the intestines, it follows that this would assist in keeping the gut barrier intact.

We know that in colitis, it is often a breach in the gut lining that sets the conditions for this disease to occur (30). Not only that, but specific colonies of inflammatory microbes then take the opportunity to develop within the gut, making the problem worse.

Intermittent fasting has been shown to reverse colitis progression in animal models (31). The authors concluded that these effects were observed because fasting restored gut barrier function and promoted a healthier microbiome.

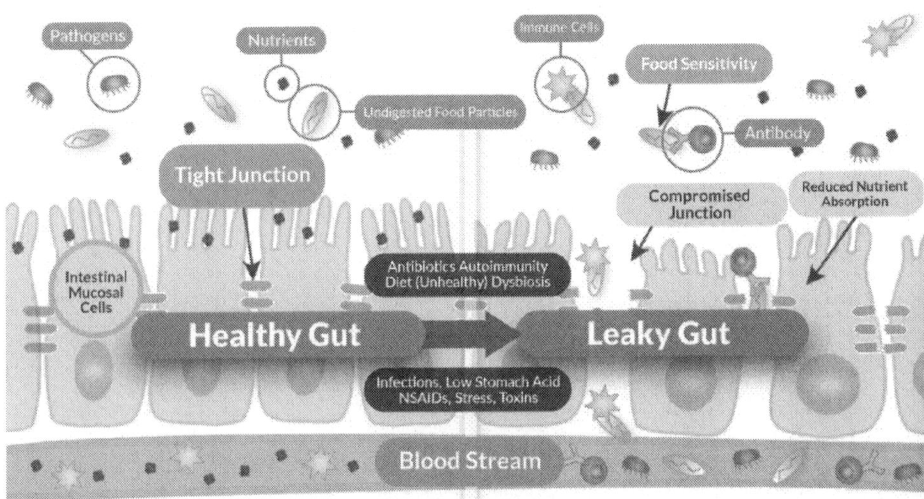

4. Increases Microbiome Diversity and Healthy Bacteria

When it comes to having a healthy gut, having a diverse array of flora is just as important as having plenty of good bacteria. Certain strains of bacteria have been shown to fight off bad bacteria and keep the gut healthy.

Fasting has been shown in several studies to improve the number of beneficial bacteria in the digestive tract.

A 2019 review on Ramadan fasting studies showed that daily fasting increased beneficial bacteria, reduced obesity, and improved blood lipids (32).

The authors of this study also noted that when people returned to their normal diet, there was a return to an unfavorable microbiome balance.

More specifically, fasting has been shown in Ramadan studies to increase the amount of *Akkermansia muciniphila, Faecalibacterium prausnitzii* and *Bacteroides fragilis* bacteria. These 3 strains of bacteria are considered by many microbiome researchers to be strong predictors of metabolic health. In fact, low levels of these bacteria are associated with metabolic disorders such as type 2 diabetes.

Another beneficial adaptation of having these bacteria is that they strengthen the integrity of the intestinal lining. This is a great benefit for anyone who has dealt with leaky gut issues.

This indicates the importance of a fasting lifestyle as well as choosing foods that further promote a healthy microbiome. This is why I love using plenty of fermented vegetables, which are rich in a diverse array of bacterial species in my meals.

Digestive Issues That May Improve with Fasting

Considering that fasting improves GI health in so many ways, many people find it helpful in healing from a number of digestive diseases. Below are some common conditions people have overcome and additional helpful tips to maximize success.

1. Leaky Gut

Leaky gut is when the gut barrier become compromised and allows things through that it typically wouldn't. This could include bacteria, viruses, or undigested food particles.

Once in the body, these things cause a cascade of inflammation and immune system dysregulation.

Common symptoms of leaky gut include brain fog, mood disorders, autoimmune conditions, and fibromyalgia. If you have any of these symptoms along with gas, bloating, indigestion, and irregular bowel movements; then you likely have some degree of leaky gut.

Fasting improves leaky gut quite effectively.

Contributors to Leaky Gut That You Would Like to Avoid Include:

- Grains
- Alcohol
- Chronic Stress
- Infections
- Antibiotic Use
- Processed, Non-organic foods
- Medications

****NOTE: These things will need to be minimized for <u>any</u> gut-related disorder**

Other Strategies to Boost Leaky Gut Healing

- Drinking bone broth
- Testing for food sensitivities
- Testing for infections
- Liquid nutrition (search my website for this strategy)
- Elimination diet or 30-day carnivore diet

2. Ulcers

Ulcers are wounds that create small openings in the lining of the stomach or intestines.

Ulcers typically develop as a result of a chronic inflammatory insult to the intestinal lining such as certain medications, an infection, smoking, alcohol, and poor diet.

Intermittent fasting is a great way to give ulcers time to recover. In addition to limiting external causes listed above, there are additional strategies that can boost your body's ability to heal an ulcer.

Other Natural Strategies for Healing Ulcers

- Testing for H. Pylori Infection
- Drinking Aloe or Cabbage Juice
- Using ginger and turmeric
- Supplementing with L-glutamine
- Taking a probiotic
- Supplementing with licorice root in a form called (DGL)

3. Crohn's, Colitis, Diverticulitis

While Crohn's disease, colitis, and diverticulitis are different in pathology, they are all inflammatory diseases of the intestinal tract.

In my clinical experience, individuals with these diseases need a similar 4 step process:

1. Fasting and removing gut-irritating foods through an elimination diet
2. Introducing gut-soothing foods like bone broth, healthy fats, and anti-inflammatory herbs
3. Using gut-healing supplements like aloe, probiotics, l-glutamine, colostrum, and digestive enzymes
4. Maintaining healthy habits like daily hydration, stress reduction, exercise, fiber (in some cases people do better with no fiber), and bathroom routines

Combining regular fasting with an elimination diet is powerful for quickly lowering inflammation in the gut and providing the best opportunity for healing.

4. **SIBO**

SIBO stands for small intestinal bacterial overgrowth. As the name suggests, this is when there is an overgrowth of bacteria in the small intestine. This causes many immediate problems like gas, bloating, diarrhea, and abdominal pain.

Long-term SIBO can contribute to skin disorders, irritable bowel syndrome, inflammatory bowel diseases, food intolerances, fibromyalgia, chronic fatigue, autoimmunity, and malnutrition.

Common causes of SIBO:

- Low stomach acid production
- Infrequent bowel movements
- Intestinal nerve damage
- Diverticula (intestinal pouches)
- History of antibiotic use or chemotherapy

Fasting may potentially be one of the quickest ways to lower bacteria counts in the small intestine. Considering these bacteria thrive on fiber, depriving them of their preferred food can help.

In addition to fasting, I recommend the following for SIBO:

- Using natural antimicrobials (berberine, oregano oil, clove, black walnut, etc.)
- Reducing or eliminating fiber through a Low FODMAPS diet, GAPS diet, elemental diet, or carnivore diet
- Using soil-based spore-forming probiotics 30–60 days after following the elimination phase with the antimicrobials.

Fasting has a wide-range beneficial impact on the digestive tract. This makes it an effective option for healing many types of digestive disorders. As you might have noticed, there are several other strategies that are helpful in healing digestive diseases that seem to overlap.

These include things like limiting dietary insults, optimizing digestion, hydrating well, exercising regularly, and using supplements if necessary. On my website, drjockers.com, I have written extensively on natural healing from different types of digestive challenges. I also have an amazing Digestive Health Program and a health coaching team to assist in your journey.

Autoimmune Disease

Autoimmune diseases have exploded in the last decade. According to the National Institute of Environmental Health Sciences, autoimmune disease affects over 24 million people in the US.

When autoimmunity occurs, a once healthy immune system can begin to attack healthy cells, tissues, or organs. This weakens the body, increases your chance of serious infection, and can eventually become life threatening in many cases.

Examples of diseases caused by autoimmunity include:

- Type 1 Diabetes
- Lupus
- Hashimoto's Thyroiditis
- Inflammatory Bowel Disease
- Multiple Sclerosis
- Celiac Disease
- Rheumatoid Arthritis
- Psoriasis and Psoriatic Arthritis

While the exact cause of autoimmunity is unknown, most health professionals agree that we must consider interactions between the environment and our genetics. We know now that genes can turn themselves on and off depending on if we eat healthy, are chronically stressed, are exposed to trauma, and a number of other factors.

While the generally held medical consensus is that there is little that can be done about these conditions, fasting and elimination dieting have produced incredible results in many cases.

Potential Causes

Through my experience working with people who have various types of autoimmune disease, I see the same tendencies over and over again.

There seems to be a connection between autoimmune disease and certain other types of health issues. Once we start to address the underlying health issues, we see improvements in autoimmunity as well.

While autoimmune diseases are certainly very complex and there is much to learn, there is also plenty we can take control of in our own lives to improve this condition.

1. **Inflammation of the Intestinal Tract**

   The intestinal tract seems to be one of the most common underlying catalysts for autoimmune disease. Whenever I get someone with an autoimmune condition, they almost always have digestive issues.

   Chronic inflammation in the intestinal tract will eventually lead to a compromised gut barrier. When this occurs bacteria, viruses, and undigested food can slip into the blood stream and create a cascade of immune activity that creates chronic inflammation.

   I believe this is the basic foundation for many autoimmune diseases and research is starting to take this into account (33). Below are some of the common causes of intestinal inflammation.

   Infections

   Your gut houses most of your immune system. Eating a poor diet, a history of antibiotic use, and chronic stress can alter your microbiome and predispose you to chronic infection.

   This can include harmful bacteria, viruses, and parasites that constantly inflame and damage your intestinal lining.

   In fact, the Epstein Barr Virus (mono) has been linked to autoimmunity and research is identifying how acute infections can lead to long-term autoimmune conditions (34).

Food Sensitivities

Consuming foods you are sensitive to can also create chronic inflammation in the gut and lead to the conditions for autoimmunity to occur.

While food allergies are very apparent, food sensitivities are low-grade inflammatory responses that you might not even know are occurring until you cut certain foods out of your diet or perform a lab test.

Over time, food sensitivities create damage to the gut lining, disruption of the microbiome, and symptoms like fatigue, brain fog, skin issues, and digestion problems. Common food sensitivities include gluten, dairy, sugar, eggs, legumes, nuts, seeds, and nightshades.

This is why I recommend performing an elimination diet or testing for food sensitivities along with fasting to optimize healing. The more sensitive you are to health challenges, the more restrictive you will likely need to be with your diet.

For the most sensitive individuals I would combine fasting with a carnivore or elemental diet.

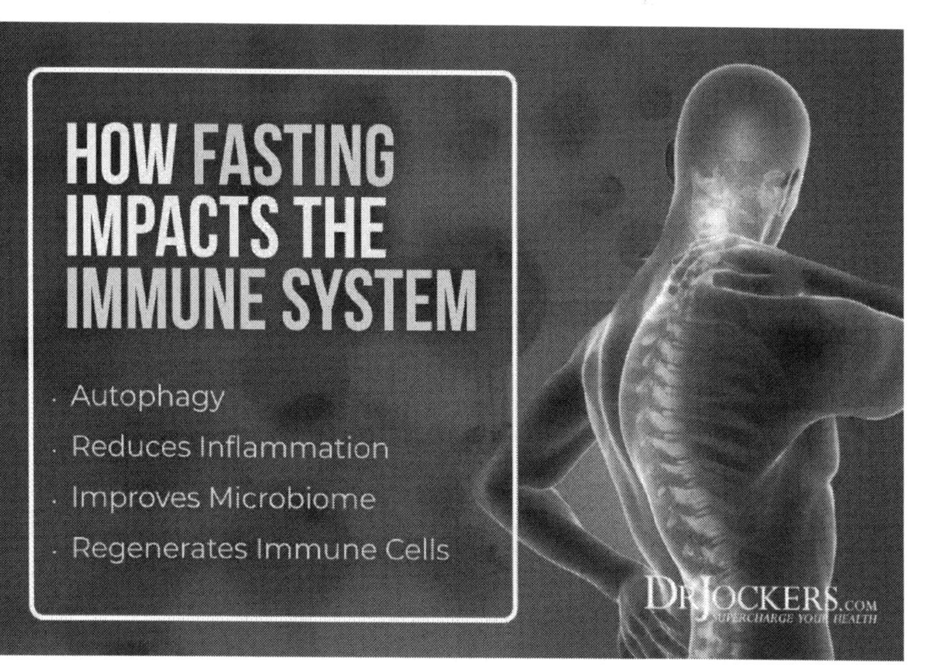

2. **Chronic Stress**

The stress response is a very primal and useful mechanism in the human body that once allowed us to avoid being killed by predators. When we go into a stress response, the body prioritizes only things that aid in immediate survival.

Unfortunately, good digestion isn't something that makes the cut. This means if you are chronically stressed, your digestion will suffer and so will your gut.

Chronic stress also makes people more likely to engage in unhealthy palliative behaviors like eating processed foods, staying up late, not exercising, and smoking.

3. **Exposure to Toxins**

Toxins are unavoidable. While modern developments have improved our lives in many ways, we've also created many toxic compounds that are not so great for the body. We are exposed to toxins in everything from the air we breathe, body care products, tap water, plastic, non-organic foods covered in pesticides, and so on.

While our bodies are mostly built to handle this toxic burden, genetics largely determine how much we can handle and individuals.

Too much exposure based on your physiology can overwhelm detoxification pathways, weaken immunity, and contribute to autoimmunity (35).

Some of the culprits I often notice in people I work with are mold or mycotoxins, heavy metals and pesticides in non-organic foods. Once we address these issues, we start to see health improvements.

4. **Nutrient Deficiencies**

Nutrient deficiencies will cause the immune system to function poorly while also decreasing your ability to detoxify properly. This will certainly contribute to autoimmunity.

Nutrients needed for a healthy immune system include:

- Magnesium
- Vitamin C
- Vitamin D
- Zinc
- B Vitamins
- Glutathione
- Selenium

Benefits of Fasting for Autoimmunity

Fasting along with a nutrient-dense diet and good hydration will address most factors that contribute to autoimmune disease (that we know of). This is a rapid-fire way to down regulate inflammation in the gut, improve the microbiome, and reset the immune system.

It seems that fasting windows of 48 to 120 hours produce the most profound effects when it comes to boosting the immune system and enhancing stress resistance.

Fasting Strategies for Autoimmunity

While all types of fasting will provide some benefit towards autoimmune conditions, there are methods I like to use in serious cases. The following 2 strategies are advanced strategies that I or one of my health coaches discuss with clients for maximum healing.

1. **Fasting & Elimination Diet**

   An elimination diet is designed to eliminate common food sensitivities and quickly reduce inflammation in the body. While it looks slightly different for everyone, you can either follow an elimination diet program or order lab testing that identifies the foods to avoid. These are both things I offer on my website.

   Fasting is a perfect companion for an elimination diet that provides a well-rounded health boost to rebalance the immune system.

2. **Fasting & Carnivore**

   If you are a very sensitive individual or prefer simplicity, the carnivore diet is the ultimate elimination diet.

   In this case you would fast and eat only animal products (minus dairy and eggs).

   Foods allowed on a carnivore diet for autoimmunity would include:

   - Grass-fed meats
   - Wild Caught Fish
   - Organ Meats
   - Collagen
   - Salt
   - Water

   This provides very rich nutrition that is easy to digest, bioavailable, and absent of compounds that can contribute to autoimmunity. While there is little research on carnivore eating, there are a growing number of testimonies from people using this method to heal chronic disease.

3. **Extended Fasting**

   Extended fasting of 48 hours or longer will create rapid shifts in the gut and immune system that make it an excellent option for supporting the body in healing autoimmune conditions.

   I have seen massive health transformations happen during extended fasting in certain cases of autoimmunity. In the next few chapters, we will be diving into how to prepare for, perform, and break an extended fast.

Neurodegeneration

As with the other diseases mentioned above, there is also an epidemic of neurodegenerative diseases. Alzheimer's and Parkinson's disease make up the vast majority of neurodegenerative disorders.

Neurodegeneration is classified by a progressive loss of neuron cells and/or myelin around nerves. It is generally accepted that these conditions get worse with time and have no cure.

It is also generally accepted that the biggest risk factor for falling victim to this disease is old age. Based on the multiple theories of ageing, we can potentially uncover lifestyle opportunities to prevent or help the body heal neurodegeneration.

It has been suggested that one of the primary mechanisms that we may be able to target in the prevention of brain degeneration is mitochondrial DNA mutations (preventing them from happening as often) and oxidative stress. These are two factors that may lead to rapid aging. Luckily, it appears fasting can both stimulate genetic repair and lower oxidative stress quite rapidly.

In Alzheimer's disease specifically, we know that there is insulin resistance within the brain (36). Similar to diabetes, the brain down regulates insulin receptors and blocks the intake of glucose. This is why Alzheimer's is now sometimes referred to as "Type 3 Diabetes" or diabetes of the brain. Perhaps this is another mechanism in which fasting can assist with healing.

Common Symptoms of Neurodegeneration Include:

- **Memory loss**
- **Forgetfulness**
- **Confusion**
- **Mood changes**
- **Loss of inhibition**
- **Anxiety**
- **Apathy**
- **Agitation**

These symptoms typically get worse with time but can be slowed with early diagnosis and medical treatment. You'll see next that there are several likely contributors to brain degeneration that can be easily managed through lifestyle as well.

Major Causes of Brain Degeneration

When it comes down to it, if you don't know what is contributing to a disease then you will not know what to change in your life to help heal it. Most people are doing things on a daily basis that are brain damaging yet they are completely unaware. Here are some of the top factors I have observed over 20 years of clinical experience.

1. Blood Sugar Imbalance

As I mentioned a moment ago, Alzheimer's disease is an almost identical pathology to diabetes in the brain. It turns out that blood sugar imbalance is actually very damaging to the brain over time.

In fact, blood sugar issues are one of the first things I suspect when someone comes to me with complaints like memory issues, brain fog, sudden irritability, cravings, and chronic fatigue. The way that most people eat favors quick, convenient, and tasty foods that create rapid blood sugar fluctuations. While eating that meal or that snack may have boosted your energy temporarily, it left you in an intense slump with no energy.

In order to sort this issue out, you need to train your body to be metabolically flexible. Fasting is the quickest way to teach your body to keep stable energy levels when no food is present. It does this by converting body fat into ketones and allowing your cells to reset their sugar burning mechanisms.

The best part about this? Your brain loves ketones!

Research on ketones and brain health has shown that an elevation of ketones in the brain was associated with: (37)

- Improved cognitive function
- Better spatial memory
- Better verbal memory
- Better energy production in the glucose-resistant brain
- Better regulation of plaque formation in the brain

While these results are promising, it was noted that following the studies many of the patients had a resurgence of symptoms after returning to a normal diet. This shows the importance of living a healthy lifestyle long term and not just for temporary alleviation of symptoms.

2. Exposure to Toxins

As we just discussed in relation to autoimmunity, toxins are unavoidable. In addition to causing chronic inflammation and dysregulation of the immune system, many toxins we face are damaging to the brain.

Some of the most common neurotoxins include:

- Mercury (Amalgam cavity fillings, certain types of fish, some vaccinations)
- Lead (Paint, tap water, soil, industrial jobs, certain cosmetics)
- Aluminum (Canned food, medications, some vaccinations, deodorant)
- Arsenic (Pesticides, herbicides, tap water)
- Alcohol
- Pharmaceutical Drugs and Recreational Drugs
- Fluoride (Toothpaste, municipal water)
- Pesticides/Herbicides/Insecticides (Non-organic produce)
- Artificial Sweeteners (Aspartame, Acesulfame Potassium, Splenda).
- MSG (Processed foods)
- Flame Retardants (Paint, furniture, carpet, treated wood, etc.)
- Mold (Water damaged buildings, packaged foods like coffee)

Fasting and proper hydration and help you expel these toxins from your body while consuming a more whole-foods nutrition plan can help limit your exposure.

I'd also recommend regular detoxification practices like using a sauna, using a home air purification system, supplementing with a bioactive carbon or activated charcoal, and exercising.

3. Sedentary Lifestyle

Movement is incredibly important for the brain and particularly for memory. Being overly sedentary is a risk factor for memory problems, trouble learning, and cognitive decline with age.

There have been studies observing thinning of brain tissue in areas of the brain associated with memory in sedentary individuals. Additionally, being overly sedentary makes you more likely to become overweight and insulin resistant.

The solution for this is pretty straight forward... move your body often!

4. Chronic Stress & Sleep Problems

When your brain perceives stress, it wants to prepare your body to get away from it. In hunter-gatherer times, this stress response prepared our muscles to run or fight something so that we could continue to live.

In modern times, many of us are setting off this stress response as we sit at our computers. Perceived stress creates the same physiological reaction in your body as physical stress, and so your body prepares accordingly.

When you experience stress one part of your brain tells another part of your brain that it is time to release cortisol. Cortisol rapidly raises your heart rate, blood sugar, and heightens your senses in the short-term.

Bursts of cortisol are important for memory formation and overall health. Chronically elevated cortisol levels can impair memory, disrupt neuron signaling, and ultimately kill brain cells. Over time, chronic stress can cause learning problems and increase risk of brain degeneration (38).

Chronic stress often coincides with poor sleep and vice versa. Sleep deprivation is also a significant risk factor for neurodegeneration as sleep is one of the brain's most important maintenance times. Research has shown an increased risk of dementia, Alzheimer's, and other neurodegenerative disorders with sleep deprivation (39, 40, 41).

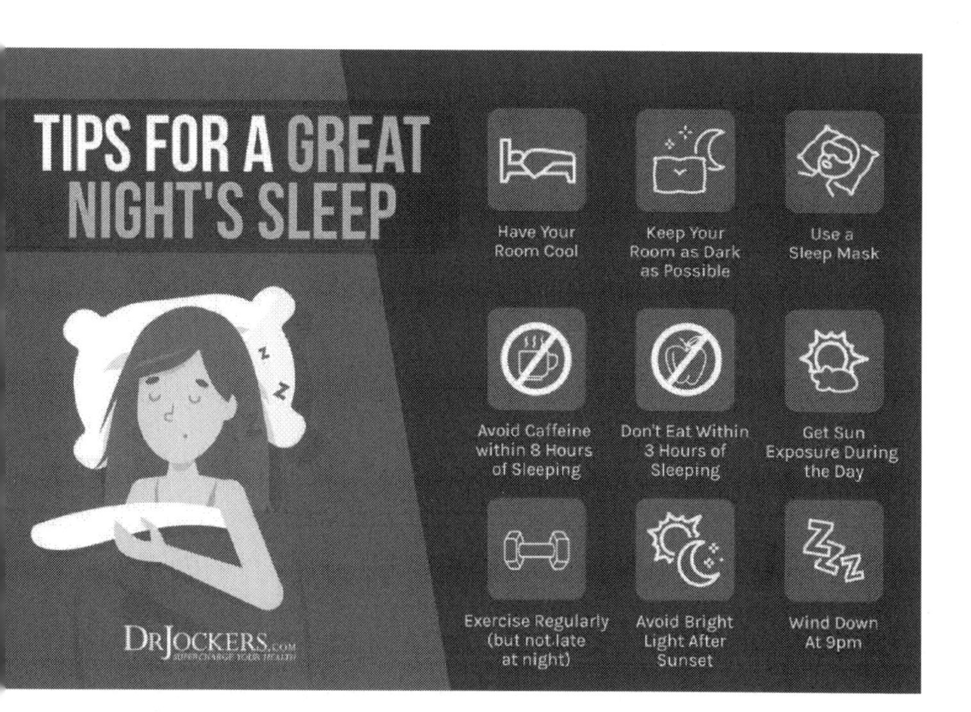

5. **Gut Infections**

   Unfavorable shifts in the microbiome can lead to chronic inflammation and negative effects on the brain. Considering the gut is where a large portion of neurotransmitters are made, keeping it healthy should be critical for brain function. Several studies reaffirm this idea by identifying the link between the microbiome and mental health (42, 43, 44, 45).

   As we've discussed several times, fasting is great for creating a healthier microbiome. Additionally, longer fasts are also great for addressing unwanted pathogens in the gut like bacteria or parasites.

Benefits of Fasting for the Brain

In addition to helping address many of the factors above, fasting has several specific mechanisms of action that boost brain health. These mechanisms generally promote a healthier brain by clearing out cells that are damaged while promoting the growth of new neurons. It is quite literally the opposite (accumulation of damaged cells and slowing of neuron growth) that classifies neurodegeneration!

1. Balances Insulin and HGH

As we have discussed already, insulin and human growth hormone (HGH) are antagonists of each other. What this means is that if insulin is elevated, HGH will be lowered. We typically see surges of HGH in the body when insulin is at its lowest points.

HGH has been recognized as a critical player in brain health. It is suspected that impairment in HGH production could play an important role in the development of Alzheimer's disease. HGH deficiency in adults is associated with impaired emotional expression, poor memory, and poor cognitive function (46).

A 2012 study found that 20 weeks of growth hormone stimulating hormone administration led to improved brain function in adults with cognitive impairments (47).

Regular fasting provides a reliable surge in growth hormone that may be able to provide similar benefits to the study mentioned above.

2. BDNF

BDNF stands for brain-derived neurotrophic factor. I know it's a mouthful but all you need to know about BDNF is that it promotes the growth of new neurons in the brain. It is essential for optimal brain function and helps to regenerate brain tissue. Sounds like something you'd want a lot of if you were at risk for neurodegeneration, right?

Higher levels of BDNF promote healthier neurons and better communication processes between cells in the brain (48). On the other hand, low levels of BDNF are linked to cognitive decline (49).

A study performed on mice found that 3 months of intermittent fasting increased BDNF levels as well as neuronal stem cells (50).

Another study published in 2019 followed 11 overweight individuals as they implemented a 6-hour time-restricted eating pattern. This study found that there was a significant elevation of BDNF in these individuals during the fasting window (51).

3. **Autophagy**

Autophagy is the body's way of recycling old cells to make room for better ones. One of the strongest stimulators of autophagy is cellular stress. When under stress, your body strives to achieve a state of homeostasis and energy efficiency. One of the ways it does this is through autophagy.

This process is extremely important for brain health as it is one of the most energy-demanding organs in the body.

Several studies have demonstrated that autophagy increases within the brain during fasting and may play a key role in improving brain health without any major side effects (52).

While daily intermittent fasts can promote autophagy, extended fasts will likely provide a higher amount. Other compounds that can boost autophagy in the brain include resveratrol and curcumin.

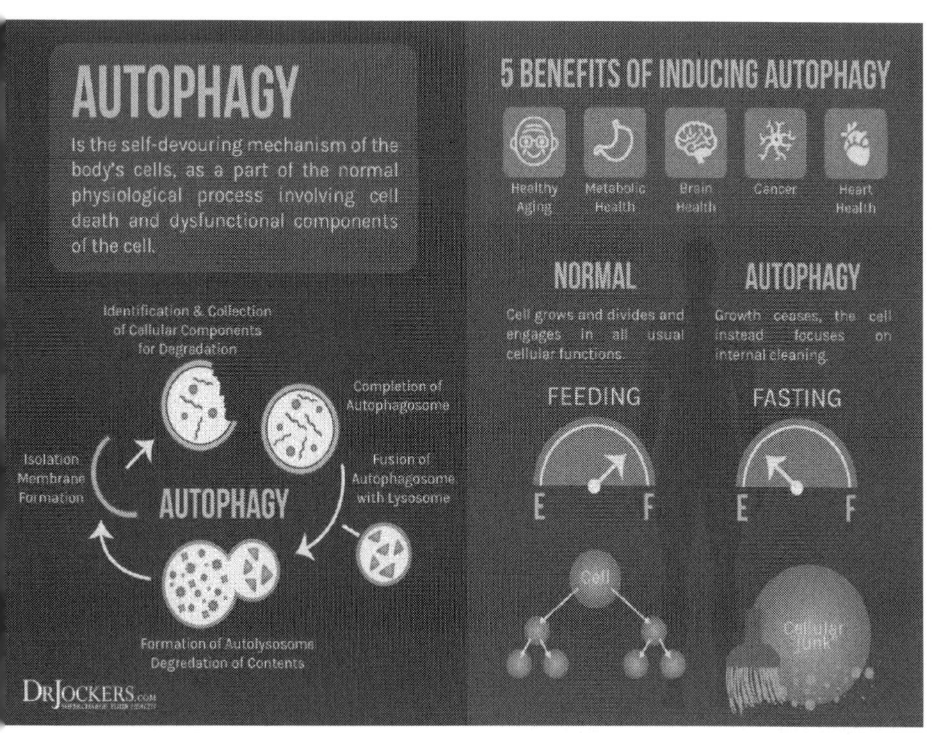

Fasting Strategies for Brain Health

In my clinical experience, I have seen a number of neurodegenerative conditions. Fasting is always a tool to consider when brain health is a concern. The following are strategies I have seen great success with.

1. **Fasting w/ Anti-Inflammatory Diet**

   One of the best ways to ensure you are supporting brain health is to fast in combination with a nutrition plan that limits toxins and blood sugar fluctuations.
   First, you'd want to be sure to eliminate garbage foods like refined sugar, gluten, grains, refined oils, processed foods, conventional dairy, and grain-fed meat.

   Next, load up on nutrient-dense foods like grass-fed meats, liver, wild-caught salmon, and organic green vegetables. Additionally, it wouldn't be a bad idea to load up on anti-inflammatory herbs and spices like turmeric, ginger, rosemary, and sage.

   Finally, you will want to have plenty of healthy fats from grass-fed butter, coconut oil, avocados, grass-fed meats, and fish.

2. **Fasting with Exercise**

   Fasting and exercise provide similar benefits on the body by rapidly depleting sugar and stressing cells. This stress causes our cells to adapt in a beneficial way. By combining exercise with fasting, you can potentially boost autophagy as well as BDNF for an even more powerful brain health response.

   It is important to do a mix of both resistance exercise and cardiovascular exercise for optimal benefits. A good goal to try and hit is 20–30 minutes of exercise, 5 days a week.

   The morning can be a great time to get your fasted exercise in! I personally perform resistance training while fasted and find I have maximum focus and energy this way.

3. **Morning Eating Window**

Sleep is also important for optimal brain health. In fact, sleep is when your brain cleans itself and performs a significant amount of autophagy.

One of the studies I discussed earlier found that when the eating window was confined to 8AM to 2PMm there were significant elevations in BDNF. This suggests that eating in the morning and fasting throughout the afternoon and into the night may be a beneficial strategy for maximizing the growth of new brain tissue.

Eating a protein-rich meal earlier in the day can also act as a circadian cue that improves sleep and stimulates the metabolism throughout the day.

4. **Extended Fasting**

Finally, and once again, extended fasting will be an important consideration for maximum autophagy and regeneration of brain tissue. Going into a deep state of ketosis and stimulating high amounts of autophagy will provide a strong anti-inflammatory effect as well as a powerful signal for healing in the brain.

Chapter 8: How to Begin Fasting

By this point in the book you may be thinking you'd like to begin fasting. It seems simple enough, just stop eating for a while, right?

While some people can go right into fasting with no issues, those dealing with illness or just getting started might want a more gradual approach to fasting.

Think of fasting similar to exercise. If you've never worked out in your life and went straight into an intense 2-hour weightlifting session right off the bat, you're probably going to be exhausted and you may even injure yourself. After having that experience it might be difficult to convince yourself to workout ever again. All you will be able to think about is how awful the experience was the first time.

Fasting can be similar. Starting with short but frequent fasts helps to condition your body and help you get metabolically fit. This chapter will be covering different strategies you can use to implement fasting into your life.

We will mainly discuss 2 strategies for implementing fasting:

1. The gradual and comfortable way
2. The quick and unpleasant way

The Gradual and Comfortable Way

The gradual way to implement fasting is designed to slowly adjust your body to increasingly longer fasting periods in preparation for an extended fast. Adapting the body to fasting over time virtually eliminates unpleasant side effects that can come along with extended fasting.

The trajectory for a gradual fasting introduction would look something like this:

Week 1 & Week 2: Eliminate sugar with a daily 12–14 hour fast

This phase is a good opportunity to get rid of any foods with added sugars. Some people choose to simply eat all of their junk food during this period while some simply dispose of or donate it somewhere else. My recommendation is to get this out of the way during week 1 so that week 2 can be focused on simply eating a low-carb whole-foods diet.

Generally, a good diet with no added sugars will be comprised of:

- Grass-fed, pastured, or wild-caught meats
- Organic vegetables
- Healthy fats
- Small amounts of low-glycemic fruits

Adding in the 12–14 hour daily fast will help adjust the body to periods without food and prepare you mentally to override your body's craving for food.

Week 3: Crescendo or cycle fasting with ketogenic refeeds

During this phase, you will stretch your fasting window to 16 hours on 2 or 3 days out of the week. Pick non-consecutive days as to not shock your system.

Additionally, the implementation of a ketogenic diet will keep your body in a fat-burning state for several days. This is a great way to prepare your body for fat-burning during a fast. The better your body is prepared for this, the easier it will be.

As a general guide, ketogenic macronutrient breakdown looks like this:

Low Carb: 5–10% of calories from net carbs (total carbs minus fiber)
Moderate Protein: 20–30% of calories from protein
High Fat: 60–80% of calories from fat

There are several ketogenic macro calculators online that can assist you in determining what your needs are.

Week 4: Daily 16–18 hour fast with ketogenic refeeds

Now that you've completed 2 or 3, 16-hour fasts in a week, you can attempt a full week of 16–18 hour fasts each day. At this point you should be very metabolically flexible with the ability to quickly shift in and out of ketosis as your body needs.

Week 5: Add a 24-hour fat fast, once per week

During week 5, pick one day out of the week to fast for 24 hours on fat. There are a number of ways to do this, but your goal is to consume no more than 40% of your normal caloric intake in fat for the day.

As we covered in Chapter 6, this would mean the average person with a daily caloric intake of 2000 calories would be allowed 800 calories of fat for that day. Ideally, you would try to consume less than this to really prepare your body for fasting.

It would be a great goal to limit yourself to 500 calories or less for improved benefits.

One of my favorite methods for fat fasting is consuming a butter coffee. The combination of caffeine and healthy fats is excellent for stimulating fat-burning.

Below is one of my go-to fat-fasting recipes (and one of the most popular on my website!):

Turmeric Fat Burning Coffee

- 2 cups of freshly brewed organic coffee
- 1 teaspoon of MCT oil or coconut oil
- 1 teaspoon grass-fed butter
- ¼ teaspoon of cinnamon
- ¼ teaspoon of turmeric
- 1 dropperful of vanilla stevia
- 1 dropperful of English toffee stevia
- A large pinch of sea salt

Other acceptable fat sources include avocado, olive oil, macadamia nuts, heavy cream, and beef tallow or suet.

Week 6: Add a 24-hour water fast, once or twice per week

Once you've comfortably adapted to all of the above, a 24-hour water fast is next.

Start with a single 24-hour fast during the week. I typically recommend doing this on a day where you have low demands and are able to rest if you need it.

This is highly individual however, as I know many people to prefer to fast on days when they have a lot of work to do. This is because some people find that their focus and productivity is highest when they are fasting.

You can then work up to adding an additional 24-hour fast in the week. As I have mentioned, I do this on Wednesday as well as Saturday as a part of my regular weekly schedule.

Once a 24-hour fast can be completed comfortably, you are ready to attempt 3–5 days of partial or water fasting!

At this point you should pretty comfortably be able to complete a 3–5-day water fast.

Alternatively, you could partake in a partial fast as we covered in Chapter 6.

In the next two chapters we will be covering what to expect, how to prepare for, and how to troubleshoot side effects on an extended fast of 3–5 days or more.

How to Know When You are Ready for the Next Step of Fasting

Sometimes it can be hard to determine if you are truly prepared for the next step in the fasting progression above. There are a number of factors that go into whether or not your body is prepared for a more advanced fasting protocol. While I do think many people can follow the trajectory outlined above, some like to go based on criteria rather than gut feeling alone.

That is why I created the **Fasting Strength Questionnaire**. I designed this tool as a way for you to determine if you need to scale up or scale down your fasting practice depending on several key factors. During each progression of your fasting journey, refer back to this questionnaire to determine if you are prepared for the next step.

Fasting Strength Questionnaire

Answer these questions to see how you are building your fasting muscle. Monitor how you feel throughout the fast after the 12-hour mark but especially so at the 4-hour window leading up to the point at which you break your fast.

Taking this quiz will help you understand your fasting fitness level and when you are ready to get more advanced.

Example: If you are doing a 16 hour fast, the peak would be hours 12–16, so pay especially close attention to how you feel during this period.

2nd Example: If you are doing an 18 hour fast, monitor closely how you feel from hour 14–18.

3rd Example: If you are doing a 24 hour fast, monitor closely how you feel from hour 20–24.

Scoring: Score your answers from left to right, 0–3 scoring

Far Left = 0 points 2nd to Left = 1 Point

2nd to Right = 2 Points Far Right = 3 points

1. **When fasting, how does your energy compare to when you are not fasting?**

   Much Worse Worse Same Better

2. **When fasting, how does your mental clarity compare to when you are not fasting?**

   Much Worse Worse Same Better

3. **When fasting, are you experiencing a lot of hunger and intense cravings?**

   All the Time Often Sometimes Very Rarely

4. **When fasting, how hard is it for you to resist food?**

   Very Hard Hard Somewhat Hard Easy

5. **When fasting, are you noticing an increase in any of these mood states compared to normal: anger, frustration, anxiety or depression?**

   All the Time Often Sometimes Very Rarely

6. **When fasting, do you feel as though you can carry out your typical daily activities?**

   Not at All Some of Them Most of Them All of Them

7. **When fasting, are you able to get a full night of sleep?**

   Rarely Some Nights Most Nights Every Night

8. **When fasting, do you wake up feeling fully rested?**

   Rarely Sometimes Usually Always

9. **When fasting, do you feel like you can typically fast longer than you originally planned?**

   Rarely Sometimes Usually Always

Total Score_______________

Fasting Fitness Level
Fasting Novice = Score of 0–16
Fasting Pro = Score of 17–21
Fasting Superhero = Score of 25+

If you scored a 17+ than you are a fasting pro and you are building your fasting muscles and are adapting to burning fat for fuel.

If you scored less than 17, you are still a Fasting Novice and it is either too early in your Fasting lifestyle to see results or your body is having trouble adapting to burning fat for fuel.

If You Are a Fasting Novice

If you are struggling to feel like you are thriving at your current fasting level, there are a number of factors to consider.

One option to consider is that you simply need more time for your body to adjust. If you feel like this is the case, then you can regress your fasting protocol by one step or simply continue at your current level until you adapt.

For example, if you are currently partaking in a daily 16-hour fast, then you may consider bumping it back to a 14-hour fast until you feel very comfortable with that. Otherwise you can remain at a 16-hour fast and implement the strategies from Chapter 11 to see if you can break your plateau.

Some options to help you adapt to fasting include:

- Performing a fat-fast with supplemental MCT oil (preferably C8 MCT oil)
- Supplementing with exogenous ketones when you begin to feel hungry or tired
- Getting some light exercise like a walk around the neighborhood or easy hike

This is a highly individual process and while some people have the physiology to push their limits, those who are very metabolically weak or fighting an illness may opt to regress their fasting strategy before taking the next step.

If you are really having a hard time with even shorter fasts, then you will likely need to pay close attention to Chapter 11 as we cover the main reasons that your body is not adapting.

If You Are a Fasting Pro

As a fasting pro, you will feel very comfortable at your current fasting level. If you are satisfied with the results you are achieving from this current fasting level, then you may choose to remain there.

If you feel comfortable at your current fasting level but are not quite satisfied with the results you are achieving, then it may be time to take the next step.

For example, if your current fasting level is a daily 16-hour fast and you would like to accelerate fat loss, then you would consider doing OMAD (one meal a day) or implementing some 24-hour fasts into your weekly schedule.

If You Are a Fasting Superhero

If you are progressing very smoothly through the fasting protocols with no side effects, then your body is likely highly adapted for fasting.

If you are one of these individuals, you may consider reasonably pushing your limits with some extended fasting or a slightly quicker progression through the fasting protocols.

This could mean spending only a few days on each progression or even skipping a level entirely.

As a health professional, my recommendation is to spend at least a week at each level to ensure a smooth progression into longer fasts.

If you reach a point where your score drops down into the **Fasting Pro** classification, then you may consider settling at that level or regressing slightly depending on your goals and daily performance requirements.

As I mentioned earlier in Chapter 5, my personal weekly routine looks like this:

- Daily 16–18-hour fasts
- 24-hour fasts on 2 days of the week (Wednesday and Saturday)
- Ketogenic nutrition during the week
- Higher carb re-feed on Sunday

This is a protocol that I have progressed myself into over several years. I closely monitored my mental and physical performance and made small tweaks over time to find what makes me the healthiest and most productive.

I do acknowledge, however, that not everyone is like me and may prefer to jump straight in to extended fasting and reverse engineer their ideal protocol from there. If you are willing to endure some discomfort in pursuit of accelerated results, then this approach may resonate with you.

The Uncomfortable Way to Start Fasting: Extended Fasting

While I do believe that just about everyone can benefit from an extended fast at some point in their lives. My general recommendation is that most people will fare better with slow and diligent progression of fasting protocols until they have built their fasting muscles to handle longer periods with ease.

This is simply due to the fact that jumping straight into extended fasting can be very uncomfortable and will easily turn most people off from fasting at all.

For those who don't mind enduring some discomfort, jumping straight into extended fasting may be their preferred method. Some proponents of fasting actually recommend beginning to do fasting this way. There is some logic as to why. Beginning your fasting journey with an extended fast of 48–72 hours will very quickly do several things like:

1. Break mental barriers and self-limiting beliefs around fasting
2. Quickly shift the body into a state of ketosis and forced adaptation to fasting
3. Rapidly promote autophagy
4. Allow an abrupt therapeutic period for the digestive tract to heal
5. Allow for a quicker adaptation to longer periods of fasting

While this will allow you to acquire the benefits of fasting much more quickly, you are also more likely to experience side effects like:

- Extreme hunger (although temporary, can be very unpleasant)
- Fatigue
- Unpleasant mood
- Headaches
- Dizziness
- Muscle cramps
- Digestive upset when re-feeding
- Constipation

- Re-feeding syndrome – a potentially fatal fasting side effect that is rare and can be easily controlled

Luckily, these side effects are much more common during the adaptation to fasting and quickly subside with continued fasting periods. Also, as we will go into detail in Chapter 11, many of these side effects can be remedied or avoided completely with proper planning.

At the end of the day, how you decide to implement fasting into your life is up to you. You can take the slow and diligent approach to minimize the unpleasant aspects of fasting, or you can go all-in with an extended fast for accelerated benefits.

As a clinician, I like the slow and controlled approach as this allows me to monitor for side effects and adjust the protocol if needed. This is especially important for very sick individuals who tend to struggle with a wide range of symptoms on a daily basis.

My coauthor, Michael, on the other hand, is a jump-in-head-first kind of guy and started out of the gates with a 5-day water fast! He admits this was a very difficult intro to fasting but found that, once he reached day 3, he adapted and completed the remainder of the fast with relative ease.

Chapter 9: What to Expect on a 5 Day Fast

Embarking on an extended fast can be pretty nerve-wracking. Especially if it is your first time. I have found that what helps people feel confident as they proceed through their fast is knowing what is happening within the body and what to expect on each day.

That is why I wrote this chapter, to prepare you mentally for the massive changes that are about to occur within your body. We are going to write out a 5-day timeline of exactly how the body reacts to a 5-day fast and even pinpoint what symptoms you may experience so that you know what to do if they come up.

That being said, remember that how you feel during a 5-day fast will differ based on a number of factors including:

- Your previous fasting experience
- Your metabolic health
- Your previous diet
- How much body fat you have
- Your previous exposure to toxins
- Your current health status

As we consider these factors, let's lay out what a 5-day fasting experience may look like.

Day 1

Days 1 and 2 out of a 5-day fast will likely be the most challenging. This is where the biggest metabolic shift occurs as your body burns away the remaining glycogen in your muscles and liver. After these stores have been depleted, this is the signal to your body to begin reaching for stored body fat for energy instead. This is when you enter a state of ketosis.

Days 1 and 2 will also be when there will be the biggest difference between those who are experienced with fasting and those starting for the first time.

Depending on how adapted you are to fasting or being in a state of ketosis, you may begin to enter mild ketosis toward the end of day 1.

If you follow the "comfortable" fasting method I detailed in Chapter 8, then day 1 will likely be pretty easy. This is because the body has been adapted to fasting and can shift into ketosis very efficiently.

If your body is well adapted to fasting, then your body will begin to activate autophagy after 16–24 hours.

For those who decide to jump straight into an extended fast with little previous fasting experience, they may experience symptoms of low blood sugar. These symptoms would include fatigue, hunger, trouble focusing, irritability, increased urination, and trouble sleeping.

Generally speaking (because there are exceptions) they will also not achieve as deep of a state of ketosis or enter autophagy quite as quickly. These changes will likely occur mostly on day 2 for non-experienced fasters.

Day 1 Side Effects

Below are common symptoms you may experience on Day 1. While they can be unpleasant, they are normal and not any reason for concern. As I have mentioned, if you have conditioned your body to fasting already, these symptoms will be very mild or non-existent.

Fatigue

Fatigue happens somewhere between your blood sugar dropping and the shift into ketosis. When you are not adapted to fasting, this transition happens slowly and results in low energy. You are experiencing the effects of low blood sugar as your body figures out how to burn fat as energy instead. When the body makes the shift into ketosis, energy levels usually stabilize or even become higher than before.

Irritability, Headaches, and Trouble Focusing

As you adapt to ketosis, your brain can experience periods of hypoglycemia. Low blood sugar in the brain can cause brain fog, mental lethargy, depression, and irritability. Hypoglycemia in the brain may also cause headaches.

Hunger & Cravings

If you are like most people, you have eaten at the same times every day for your entire life. Your body adapts to this and creates hormonal rhythm to mirror your habits. More specifically, the hormone ghrelin is released when the stomach is empty or around times of the day that you have conditioned yourself to eat.

When you first start fasting, you will experience sudden bouts of hunger as your body has learned to expect food. While this can be uncomfortable, it is not dangerous, and you are not starving... You are just fighting a habit that has been engrained in your physiology.

Increased Urination

As you metabolize glycogen and your insulin levels begin to drop, your body will begin to retain less water. Additionally, you will likely be drinking slightly more water than usual. This will naturally result in you needing to pee more.

Sleep Problems

Fasting slightly raises your cortisol levels which can raise energy levels. Additionally, hypoglycemia can make sleeping difficult. Once in a state of ketosis, many people actually report sleeping quite well. Initially, it can be helpful to increase magnesium intake to assist with relaxation. You may also consider using melatonin and anti-stress herbs like ashwagandha.

Day 2

Day 2 is generally the toughest day of the fast for adapted and non-adapted fasters. Oftentimes, day 2 will bring about the same continued symptoms of day 1 – minus the hunger. If you do experience hunger, that doesn't mean there is anything wrong with you. It just means your body is still adapting.

On day 2 it is still common to experience some fatigue, irritability, headaches, and trouble focusing. This is the time during the fast when you will need to face the biggest mental barriers. While the experience of Day 2 may be temporarily unpleasant, getting past this hump is usually the hardest part of the entire fast.

It is common that once people make it past the 48-hour mark of their fast, they experience high levels of energy and mental clarity that make the rest of the fast much easier. Stick in there!

Day 2 Symptoms

In addition to the symptoms that are common on day 1, there can be an increase in fatigue, brain fog, and irritability. This emotional instability can make it very easy to convince yourself to break the fast early. This is why day 2 is typically the most difficult as you push yourself through.

Other symptoms that can sometimes occur on day 2 are:

Tongue Changes

Some people report that their tongue will take on a white thrush to it as they shift deeper into ketosis. In more rare cases, the tongue can take on a yellow or black color. This is a build-up of keratinized skin cells on the tongue that are typically rubbed off with normal consumption of food and are not dangerous. If you'd like you can use a tongue scraper to remove this top layer of dead skin cells.

Cold Fingers and Toes

When fasting, your brain detects that there are no calories entering the body. After 24 hours, your brain will slow down your metabolism via thyroid hormone to improve energy efficiency. This results in less energy getting turned into heat. This results in a slightly lower body temperature and, more noticeably, cold hands and feet.

Rashes

While it is rare, some people experience rashes on day 2 of a fast. Because the microbiome of the digestive tract is directly tied to skin health, it is likely that changes in the gut are influencing the development of rashes short-term.

When fasting, many types of microbes in the gut can starve off and release toxic byproducts as they die. These byproducts elicit a histamine reaction within the skin that cause inflammation and rashes. While unpleasant, this response may be a sign that you are going through a healing response.

Day 2 Health Effects

While there are many health benefits that happen during the first 24 hours of a fast, day 2 is when they intensify greatly. These health benefits experience a steep rise on day 2 and continue to increase with each successive day of the fast. There is a law of diminishing returns, however, as the benefits seem to level off around day 5 as well. This makes a 5-day fast an excellent goal.

Some of the changes occurring in the body on day 2 include:

A Surge in Human Growth Hormone

As you shift into a deeper state of ketosis, the body releases growth hormone to preserve muscle mass and stimulate fat-burning. HGH also boosts the immune system and promotes bone density.

Increases Cellular Autophagy

Your body will begin to break down and recycle old and weak cells, recycling the components to help the formation of new more efficient cells. One of the greatest benefits of this is mitochondrial biogenesis, the development of more efficient mitochondria.

Stem Cell Proliferation

Along with autophagy, the body creates new white blood cells, repairs the intestinal lining, and boosts stem cells within the joints to assist with the repair of damaged tissues.

Changes in the Microbiome

The absence of food and fermentable fibers starves unwanted microbes in the digestive tract to allow the proliferation of healthier species.

Optimization of Hormones

Thyroid hormones, insulin, estrogen, testosterone, and several others are vital for overall health. During a fast there is downregulation of receptor sites for many of these hormones. This makes your body more sensitive to these hormones and makes your hormone response much more efficient. Increasing insulin sensitivity to improve blood sugar is a prime example of this.

Day 3

Day 3 is what many people consider being "over the hump". This is when the body has shifted into ketosis and is burning ketones for energy. Keep in mind that if you did not prepare your body for the 5-day fast by partaking in shorter fasts or a ketogenic diet, then this may take longer for your body.

For many people, however, Day 3 is when energy levels begin to rise and the uncomfortable symptoms from days 1 and 2 subside.

If you still experience some fatigue or brain fog, you are still adapting, and this is a normal feeling.

Day 3 Health Effects

On day 3 you will experience an increase in growth hormone, autophagy, and stem cell production. Additionally, many people report that certain types of pain in the body begin to diminish and become less noticeable.

It'd be a great idea to track your blood ketone levels to monitor whether or not you are shifting into a deeper state of ketosis.

While urine ketone strips are readily available and easy to use, they are not necessarily an accurate measurement of your current level of ketosis.

In addition to blood ketone measurements, breath ketone monitors are also a great tool.

The average person will see a rise in ketone levels on days 3 and 4 that coincide with heightened energy levels and mental clarity.

If you search DrJockers.com for "ways to measure ketone levels" you will find an in-depth article that covers how to measure ketones and my favorite measurement devices.

Gauging Your Day 3 Ketosis Adaptation

Day 3 is a great time to get an idea of how adapted your body is to fasting. My recommended way of doing this is determining your Glucose Ketone Index or GKI.

The GKI is a measurement that the prominent metabolism researcher Dr. Thomas Seyfried devised to measure the response of tumors to fasting and ketosis (1).

On a more general level, the GKI is a great way to see how well your body is adapting to using ketones as an energy source over glucose.

A good indication of nutritional ketosis is a GKI between 1:1 and 4:1. Being within this range is considered nutritional ketosis and is considered a positive adaptation.

In the case of cancer, however, a deeper state of ketosis is recommended, and you would want to see a GKI closer to 1:1. This indicates your ketone levels are much higher in relation to glucose. As we discussed in Chapter 7, burning ketones as a primary fuel source places cancer cells at a metabolic disadvantage and gives the immune system the upper hand in wiping them out.

So, what does a 1:1 GKI look like in everyday glucose and ketone measurements?

For most people you are looking for:

A blood glucose measurement in the 60's

A blood ketone level of 3.0 mmol/L or higher

To reach these therapeutic levels, the average person would need to water fast for 4–5 days.

To calculate your GKI, use the following equation:

GKI = (Blood Glucose/18) / Blood Ketones

In order, you divide your blood glucose number by 18 first. Once you have that number, you divide it by your blood ketone levels.

Dr. Seyfried has observed the 1:1 GKI to me most effective for shrinking tumors. This is likely due to high levels of autophagy and low levels of insulin making it difficult for glucose to gain entry into cancer cells.

Other tips for keeping a low GKI include:

- Reducing stress
- Engaging in low-level activity like regular walks in the sunshine
- Improving Vitamin D levels through sun exposure
- Refeeding with ketogenic meals
- Optimize your sleep

Day 4

As we just discussed, days 4 and 5 are where ketone levels will reach the highest levels and bring you close to a GKI of 1:1.

This is where autophagy, ketone levels, and mental clarity should reach its peak as well.

Personally, days 4 and 5 are my most productive days as I feel light and energized. Most people report having very little desire to eat on these days. While some people will still be dealing with the emotional pull towards food, hunger and strong cravings are typically absent.

If you feel like you are still struggling to adapt at this stage, there are common reasons for this including:

- Stress
- Constipation
- Release of toxicity from fat stores
- Poor hydration or electrolyte levels

In certain cases, I recommend certain supplements to assist with the healing processes that are taking place. We will go more into this in Chapter 11 where we discuss troubleshooting common challenges people face when fasting.

As a brief precursor, here are some tips for helping your body through this point in the fast:

- For stress – Adaptogenic herbs and Unsweetened magnesium
- For a low GKI – Exogenous ketones
- For constipation – Oxygen-based intestinal cleanser
- For detoxification – A toxin binder that reaches the cellular level such as bioactive carbon
- To further support detoxification and mental clarity – Hydrogen-enriched water or a reduced, acetylated or liposomal form of glutathione

Day 5

Day 5 is when most fasting benefits reach their peak. This is when growth hormone, stem cells, and autophagy are at their highest.

The end of Day 5 is great time to slowly reintroduce food as your body has now been breaking down old tissues for several days and stem cells are ready for nourishment so they can optimize tissue repair.

Similar to day 4, most people feel great on day 5 and do not have strong food cravings.It is at this point where some people decide if 5 days is enough or that they want to extend the fast even longer.

While fasting longer than 5 days still has benefits, fasting for longer than 5 days may start to lower lean body mass.

If you are a lean individual, such as myself, I like to stay in the 4–5 day range to optimize healing benefits without sacrificing muscle.

If you have higher amounts of body fat and want to continue on your fast, you can do so as long as you are feeling stable.

I have witnessed several individuals take on fasts for 11, 30, or even 40+ days and seen tremendous benefits. Approaching these much longer fasts will require diligent body monitoring, hydration with minerals, and potential supplementation of micronutrients.

Breaking the Fast

At the 5-day mark of a fast, your digestive system has been shut down for some time and needs a gentle reintroduction of foods to get it readjusted.

Take the amount of days you fasted, divide it by 2, and create a food reintroduction schedule that starts with easy to digest foods and gradually adds in things like meat, eggs, and raw vegetables.

For example, if you fasted for 5 days then you'd want 2.5 days to work your way up to that juicy grass-fed steak you've been dreaming about.

A 2.5-day food reintroduction plan would look like this:

> **Day 1: Protein Shakes with berries, fruits, green juices, bone broth, coconut water kefir, slow-cooked or pressure-cooked soups**
>
> **Day 2: Add in <u>small amounts</u> of fish, slow-cooked meats with bone broth, and fermented vegetables**
>
> **Day 3: Return to more solid foods including healthy fats, vegetables, starches, and meat**

For shorter or longer fasts, use this same principle. A 3 day fast would need a 1–1.5 day reintroduction period while an 8–10 day fast would need 3–5 days. This is also individual specific so test what works best for you and create your ideal fasting schedule.

How Often Should You Do an Extended Fast?

How often you perform an extended fast depends on a number of factors. These are the generalized guidelines I go by.

Most people do great in the 4–5 day range, so this is a good place to start. If you are dealing with a lot of excess body fat and debilitating inflammatory disorders, you might consider approaching the 8–10 day window. Alternatively, you could also perform 4–5 day fasts more frequently. For example, these individuals might consider performing a 4–5 day fast once a month or an 8–10 day fast every other month.

For added benefits, these individuals would also want to partake in some type of intermittent fasting strategy like a cycle fast, strong fast, or alternate day fast.

For lean individuals, as I alluded to already, 3–5 days is great to achieve health benefits without losing body weight unnecessarily. For lean individuals with debilitating chronic inflammatory conditions, you could perform a 3–5 day fast every 8–12 weeks.

This stimulates profound changes in the body over a 6–8 month period. These individuals would likely notice having a much easier time fasting each time as the body becomes healthier.

HOW LONG AND HOW OFTEN TO FAST FOR BEST RESULTS

This is a very personal thing but for best results use the following chart. In general, the more weight you have to lose and the more inflammation and chronic disease manifestation your body has experienced, the longer and more frequent you can fast for best results.

Body Type	Health Goal	Duration	Frequency
Thin/Lean	Reduce Inflammation/ Chronic Disease	3-5 Days	Every 8-12 Weeks
Normal Wt	Reduce Inflammation/ Chronic Disease	4-7 Days	Every 6-8 Weeks
Overweight	Lose Weight/ Inflammation/ Chronic Disease	5-10+ Days	Every Month

If you aren't battling a chronic disease or want to aggressively reduce inflammation and rebuild your body than doing a longer fast 1 or 2 times per year is all I would normally recommend.

This is not meant to treat any specific condition and please consult your health care practitioner before beginning a fasting regimen

DRJOCKERS.COM

Chapter 10: Preparing for Your Extended Fast

So, let's say you are planning on taking on a 3–5 day water fast. Independent of which method you have decided to use to prepare your body (as discussed in Chapter 8), there are still some critical steps you will want to take to ensure your fast goes smoothly.

This chapter is oriented around the 1–2 weeks leading up to your extended fast.

Coming from a clinical perspective and working with very sensitive individuals, I like to see that most people have done the following before embarking on their first extended fast:

- A minimum of 2–3 weeks of intermittent fasting with ketogenic diet
- Ideally the individual has completed several 24-hour fasts with relative ease to ensure they are adapted to fasting
- If you are on a tight time window, try to complete at least 2, 20–24 hour fasts in the 1–2 weeks leading up to your extended fast

Fasting is a muscle, the more you work it, the more efficient your body gets at it. This is why someone who does not train their body for a longer fast may have a significantly different experience than someone who has slowly built up to it over time.

That being said, the body is able to adapt rather quickly when the stimulus is strong enough. If your health situation requires immediate and strong action, these steps will still help your body prepare for an extended fast even if you have no prior fasting experience.

Strategy #1: Reduce Your Schedule Demands

Being overly stressed will significantly throw off your fasting resilience. This is because, when you are stressed, hormones become erratic, blood sugar dysregulates, and it can become quite easy to talk yourself out of fasting.

Take some time to plan out your schedule so that you can spend a little more time relaxing than usual. If you have a very demanding job, this is a great time to take a vacation or work a limited schedule. This is also a great time to begin a mindfulness practice that teaches you to control your stress response. This could be anything from short 10-minute breathing exercises (Heart Math is a great one), sitting quietly in the sun, or engaging in a low-demand movement practice.

Taking time to heal your body is critical. You can re-earn money lost but you can't regain time. Give yourself permission to relax and take in the full benefits of this therapeutic time in your life. The people in your life need you to be healthy just as much as they need your service.

This is especially important for your first fast as it will likely be your most challenging. As you become experienced with longer fasts you might actually find that you have a higher stress tolerance and greater mental output when you are fasting. If you feel like you are at this point, then it may actually be beneficial for you to stay busy and keep your mind focused on your goals.

If you have read this section and you think it is impossible for you to reduce your workload for an extended fast, then it may not be the best time for you to start an extended fast. Either that or you need to take a vacation more than anyone else!

Strategy #2: GIVE YOURSELF PERMISSION TO REST

Although I already stated this in the previous section, it is so important that I had to bring it up again in its own section.

You MUST give yourself permission to rest and heal. Everyone who depends on you, depends on you taking care of yourself as well. In our society, people seem to get stuck in this idea that if we're not constantly busy, then we're not getting anything done or we're losing value.

Being productive and being busy are very different things. Taking the time to rest and rejuvenate your body is extremely productive. Gaining your health and vitality back is paramount to your productivity in every other aspect of your life as well.

Especially if this is your first fast. Go out of your way to take a break and give yourself permission to relax and take in all of the powerful benefits of a fast.

Do this knowing that when you get back to your regular work schedule, you will be a better human!

Listen to your body during this first fast. You will likely experience bouts of fatigue or irritability. This is a great time to do something relaxing that is not too mentally engaging. This could be taking an Epsom salt bath, it could be taking a nap, it could even be watching a good movie.

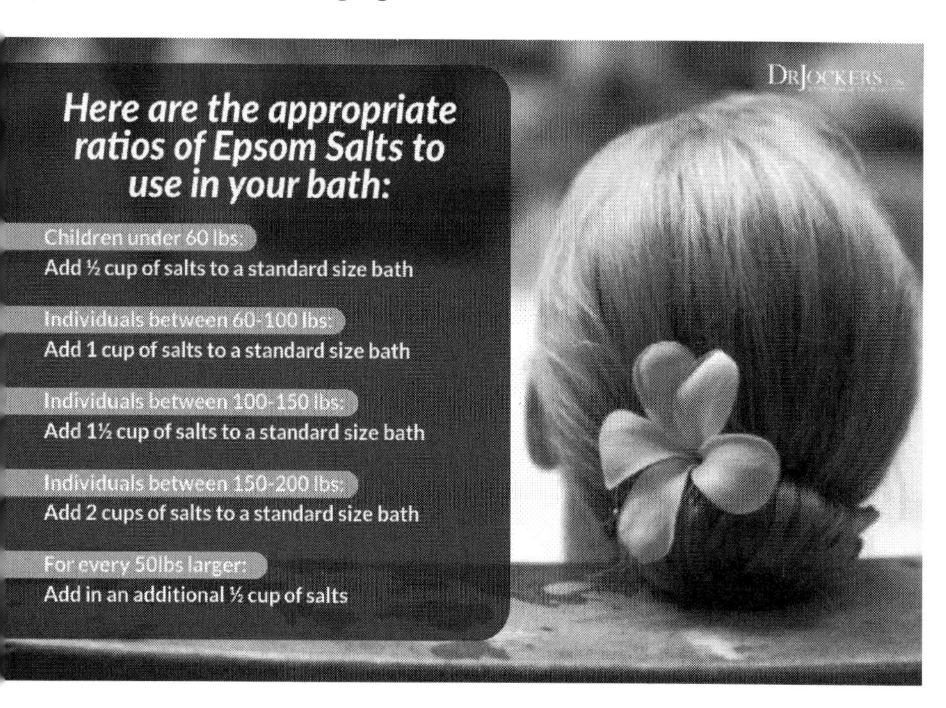

Strategy #3: Schedule a Spa Day

Continuing the theme from strategy 2, take a day and get yourself pampered. With the money you are saving by not eating for 5 days, it is a great idea to find yourself a spa and get away for one or even multiple days.

Getting a massage and using spa amenities like a sauna for short periods is a great way to relax and assist your body with detoxification. Ensure you are staying properly hydrated of course.

Let's be honest, your first extended fast may not be very enjoyable. By scheduling a spa day on day 2 or later on in the fast, you give yourself something enjoyable to look forward to and reward yourself for pushing through the discomfort.

Considering most people have some type of emotional reliance on food, they may have to face some uncomfortable emotions as they take away that crutch. Getting pampered is a great way to deal with those emotions while keeping on track with your goals.

Strategy #4: Avoid People Who Will Not Support Your Efforts

Chances are if you've told more than one person about your plans to fast, you've gotten at least one person look at you with their eyes popping out of their head like you're crazy...

You will always have people who think you're crazy for taking care of your health. During a time like this, it is best to just avoid being around or communicating with those people if possible.

Instead spend time with those who support your efforts or find an online fasting accountability group that you can lean on if you struggle at all.

If it happens to be that those people are close family or people you cannot avoid. It may be helpful to sit them down the week before your fast and have a heartfelt conversation about why you are choosing to undergo this process and how important their support is to you. Tell them that all you need from them is a bit of encouragement if things get tough.

On your end, when you receive the right kind of support you asked for, be sure to provide positive reinforcement to let them know that they are being helpful. Communication is very important here.

If you know you will have to deal with some negativity during your fast, take some time out of each day to express gratitude. Getting in the habit of expressing the things you are grateful for helps to ground you emotionally and make you more resilient to the negativity you may experience.

One of my favorite gratitude practices is getting a journal and writing down 3 things you are grateful for first thing in the morning and just before going to bed. There are also great phone journaling apps that can be used for this. Simply search gratitude journal on your phone's app store.

Strategy #5: Drink Water

Hydration is critical on an extended fast. As your body uses up stored glycogen in the muscles and liver, it will deplete water levels with it. Additionally, as your insulin levels drop and you approach entering into ketosis, your body will begin to excrete sodium and water.
Assist your body in this process by consuming high-quality water like reverse osmosis or bottled spring water in glass containers. Adding in a pinch of salt or making an electrolyte solution as outlined in Chapter 5. Here it is again so you don't have to flip back:

Mixed in 1 Liter of Water,

Sea Salt – ½–1 tsp (providing about 1000 mg of sodium)
Potassium chloride – ½ tsp (providing about 1600 mg of potassium)
Magnesium Glycinate – ½ tsp (providing about 200 mg of magnesium)

You would want to slowly sip on this solution throughout the day. If you are urinating very frequently or have loose bowels, then that is a sign to back off or drink plain water temporarily.

To reach the RDA amounts of each of these electrolytes, you would need to drink approximately 3 Liters of this solution.

Ideally, you will want to drink a minimum of one ounce of water per pound of bodyweight. Oftentimes, clients find it helpful to consume a gallon of water or more during a fast.

You will likely feel hungry around the times of day you regularly eat. This is because your body has adapted to a natural rhythm of eating and hunger hormones such as ghrelin will surge during these times. This is a good time to drink water to help gently stave off hunger and keep on track with your fast.

You may also find it helpful to consume herbal teas like green tea, chamomile, or ginger tea. The warm liquid can help soothe the belly and get you through your hunger.

Strategy #6: Add Some Salt

As I have touched on already, salt and electrolytes are just as important for hydration levels as water is. This is why adding some salt to your water or making the electrolyte solution above can help tremendously with keeping energy levels up during a fast.

I have had several people report to me that there is a night-and-day difference in how they feel when they fast with electrolytes versus when they only consume plain water.

If you begin to feel overly tired or dizzy during your fast, either make an electrolyte solution to sip on or simply put a big pinch of salt on your tongue and chase it down with 4–8 ounces of water and see if it helps.

Strategy #7: Get Sunshine & Ground Yourself

Sunlight is healing to body for many reasons. Depending on where you are in the world, you will get varying amounts of Infrared and ultraviolet light throughout the day.

Infrared is typically found in higher amounts during the early morning and sunset with benefits including:

- Improving skin health and appearance
- Improving muscle or joint pain
- Boosting mitochondrial energy output
- Increasing mental clarity
- Promoting relaxation

You can also get these benefits by using one of several red-light therapy panels that include the wavelengths 660nm and 850nm for optimal health benefits.

Ultraviolet light is more prominent in the middle of the day when the sun is in the middle of the sky. This is the type of light that boosts the immune system and optimizes several key hormones in the body through the generation of Vitamin D.

Using an app like DMinder is a great way to determine what the UV levels are where you live and track how long you should spend outside for optimal benefits.

Getting sun optimizes your body in many ways and assists with fat-burning to speed the transition into ketosis during your fast. Additionally, sunlight stimulates neurotransmitters that make you feel good like serotonin, dopamine, and endorphins.

If you are in the position to do so, this is a great reason to take a vacation and get out in the sun! If this is not an option for you, still take regular breaks to go outside.

In addition to getting sunlight, make sure to get barefoot contact with the ground regularly throughout your fast. Due to the electromagnetic interaction between the sun and the earth, the earth releases natural negative ions that the human body can absorb. Due to the rubber sole in modern day shoes, this healing benefit is lost.

There is some good research showing that people who regularly ground themselves feel less stress and experience lower levels of inflammation.

Strategy #8: Move, but Gently

As you fast, your body is going to be hard at work breaking down, recycling, and eliminating different types of compounds. One of the major pathways that needs to be optimized during this time is the lymphatic system.

The lymphatic system spreads throughout the body similar to your veins and arteries which circulate blood. The major difference in your lymphatic system is that it does not have a pump to promote circulation.

Instead, your lymphatic system circulates when muscles contract around it. This is why getting regular movement is great for you during a fast.

In this case, we are talking about very gentle exercise like light mobility work or walking in the sun. Something else that helps greatly with lymphatic circulation is massage! Another reason to treat yourself to a spa day.

40–60 minutes of movement is a great goal. Break this up into several movement sessions throughout the day. You can certainly do more activity than this if you are feeling up to it.

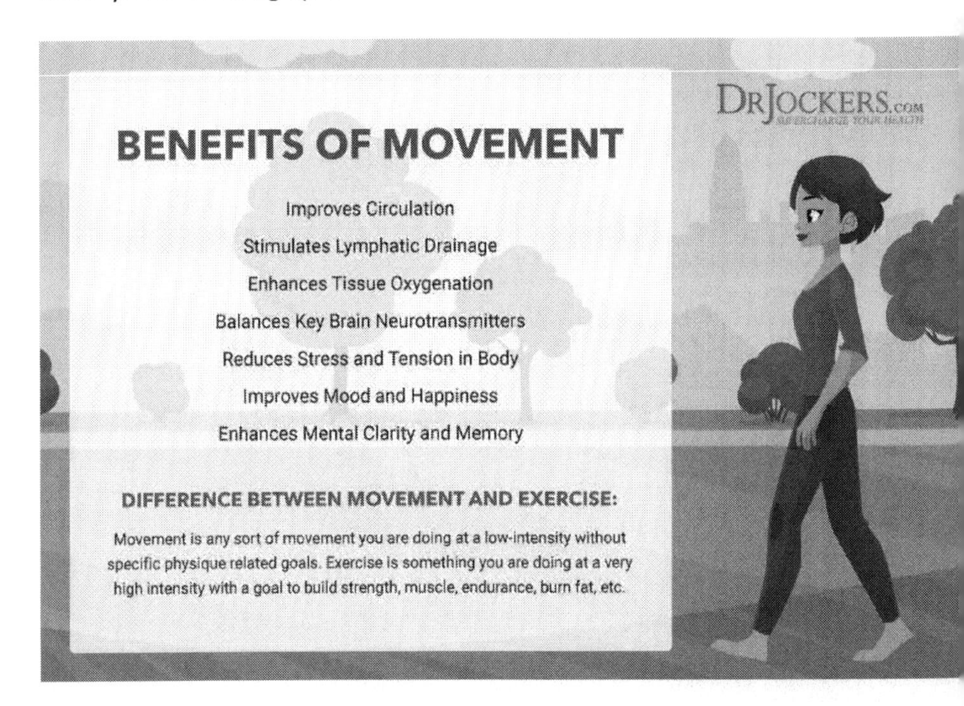

Strategy #9: Use Natural Sweeteners If Needed

Sometimes when cravings are hitting really hard and you're having a hard time staving them off, a little something sweet can go a long way. Using sweeteners like stevia that have zero calories can help boost your mood and make the more challenging parts of your fast enjoyable.

One of my go-to recommendations in this case is making a sugar-free lemonade by combining water, fresh lemon juice, and a little bit of stevia.

There are now a wide variety of stevia flavors that can curb that sweet tooth in most cases.

Other ideas I have gotten from my fasting group are:

- Lemon seltzer water with lemon lime stevia
- Iced green tea with peach or raspberry lemonade stevia
- Ginger tea with lemon stevia

Obviously, the possibilities are endless. Just ensure you purchase a brand of stevia that is not combined with regular sugar or other chemically synthesized sweeteners that are not the best for someone who is trying to be healthy.

Strategy #10: Avoid the Kitchen the Best You Can

Chances are your brain associates the kitchen with mealtime or snack time.

Have you ever walked into the kitchen with no intentions of eating only to find yourself standing in front of an open fridge snagging little bites of anything that sounds good at the moment? Yeah... everyone has.

Try to be intentional about how much time you spend in the kitchen. This will be especially important during the first 2 days of the fast as cravings will be a bit more prominent during this time.

If you have to cook for other people or are unable to avoid the kitchen, it is a good idea to have your water or herbal tea on hand to help reduce the drive to eat.

Chapter 11: Troubleshooting Fasting Challenges

You understand by now that fasting is a powerful healing tool. You also understand that it comes with its unique challenges.

At the beginning of your fasting journey, it is likely that you will run into discomfort. I challenge you to acknowledge this discomfort and face it head-on. On the other side of this discomfort is a massive amount of transformative potential.

There will likely also be times where this discomfort will lead you to stopping your fast shorter than you originally planned. I urge you to not take this as a failure. Going through this process over and over again will help you understand when you really need to break your fast or when you're just going through the regular process outlined in the last chapter.

As you get further down the path of the fasting lifestyle, you will figure out what your body responds well to. Your fasting needs will change with time so don't get too caught up in always fasting one particular way.

You will build your fasting intuition and grow into your ideal fasting routine.

In this chapter, we are specifically going to touch on some of the sensations you could experience during your fasts and ways to mitigate them for a smoother fasting experience.

Challenge #1: Dizziness, Fatigue, and Headaches

Dizziness, fatigue, and headaches are the most common fasting challenges I hear about from my coaching clients. If you are someone who is accustomed to 3 square meals a day, plus snacks, since you were born – then this is likely the feeling you experience right before you decide it's time to eat!

Many people experience this dip in energy every single day. Now think about if this is you and how many times you've engrained the thought, "Oh I'm starting to get tired and moody; it must be lunch time!".

The reality is that most people have been going through this cycle their entire lives. If you are experiencing a more intense version of this when you begin fasting, your body is likely still trying to break that subconscious pattern.

As you become adapted to fasting, your body will quickly shift into ketosis and energy levels will stabilize or even increase in many cases.

There are other factors that play into this, however.

Reasons Why This Can Happen

Dizziness, fatigue, and headaches can all occur while fasting for several reasons including:

- Low blood sugar (before ketone levels increase)
- Dehydration
- Depletion of salt levels
- Lack of movement
- Lack of sunlight
- Detoxification reactions

Luckily, dizziness and fatigue are especially common for people who are brand-new to fasting. These symptoms quickly reside as the individual becomes adapted to fasting regularly and dials in their ideal water and electrolyte intake.

How You Can Prevent or Fix It

The first strategies I go to when someone is complaining about these common symptoms are making sure that they are drinking enough water and getting enough salt. In this case, the fasting electrolyte solution detailed in Chapter 10 is something to consider.

After you hydrate well, go for a light walk in the sunshine and see how you feel. If it is an especially hot day, wait until late afternoon or early morning to do this.

This is also a great time to give yourself permission to rest. Taking a nap, laying out a blanket at the park, or laying in a hammock are all excellent restful activities.

At the end of this chapter, we will go into supplements that can help to mitigate many of the side effects from fasting as well.

Challenge #2: Constipation

Constipation can be uncomfortable and make you feel like... well... crap.

In addition to feeling backed up, having stagnant waste in your colon can contribute to dizziness, fatigue, and headaches.

This is because backed up waste can create excessive fermentation, an overgrowth of bacteria, and the release of toxic byproducts that inflame the brain.

In fact, persistent brain fog is almost always associated with gut disorder.

How You Can Prevent or Fix It

If you are someone who is prone to constipation, the following are ways to assist your body with elimination. These are especially helpful to eliminate excess waste right before beginning an extended fast.

- Ensuring optimal water and electrolyte intake
- Staying active
- Consider a colonic or coffee enema
- Supplement with a bioactive carbon to bind toxins in the colon

THE IMPORTANCE OF HEALTHY BOWEL MOVEMENTS

Having good bowel habits may be one of the most important elements in your overall health journey. Prioritize having good bowel activity each and everyday.

Healthy Bowel Movement Habits:

- Happen 1-4 Times Daily
- Moving Out All Waste From Previous Meals Within 24 hours
- Best Daily Rhythm is Early in the Morning and/or Shortly After Meals

Healthy Bowel Movement Habits:

- Reduces the Microbial Load on the Body
- Eliminates Destructive Endotoxins
- Reduces Inflammation Throughout the Body
- Helps Calm the Brain and Nervous System
- Enhances Energy and Mental Clarity
- Improves Skin Health and Natural Glow
- Reduces Chronic Pain Levels

DrJockers.com

Challenge #3: Toxic Reactions

As we just discussed, being chronically constipated is one way that your body can take on a higher toxic burden. Aside from this, many people experience detoxification reactions for another reason.

Detoxification reactions are common during fasting even in those who are not dealing with constipation. This is because we are exposed to a wide variety of toxins every day that, many of which, are stored in fat tissue.

When you begin fasting, you will undoubtedly begin to release some of these toxins as you begin to burn off body fat.

Again, luckily this is more common in the beginning stages of fasting and is easily mitigated if you plan properly.

Another, often overlooked, contributor to these toxic reactions is actually a very beneficial resetting of the gut microbiome. Fasting will begin to drastically shift the microbial balance of the gut as pathogenic bacteria and fungi begin to die off. This die off releases toxic byproducts into the digestive tract that can sometimes become absorbed into the blood stream and cause inflammatory reactions.

This reaction can be mitigated by taking activated charcoal or a bioactive carbon supplement.

How You Can Prevent or Fix It

Toxic reactions do not happen to everyone, but they are also not uncommon. The symptoms of these toxic reactions can be anything from nausea, brain fog, headaches, fatigue, chills, aches, and just about any other unpleasant feeling in the body.

The best thing you can do in this situation is bind and eliminate.

First of all, you want to do everything you can to support your detoxification pathways. This means your bowels are moving, you are properly hydrated, and you are stimulating your lymphatic system through regular exercise.

Next, the best thing you can do when you are already dealing with this reaction is to take a bioactive carbon that is able to absorb into the bloodstream and bind to these toxins so they cannot interfere with regular body processes. I carry several great bioactive carbons on my online DrJockers.com store.

Finally, you must understand that rapid changes are occurring within the body. While sometimes unpleasant sensations can occur, this is a part of the body's adaptation process. The best option you have is to support your body as it goes through these changes for optimal benefits. In a moment, we will discuss supplements that can help you in this process.

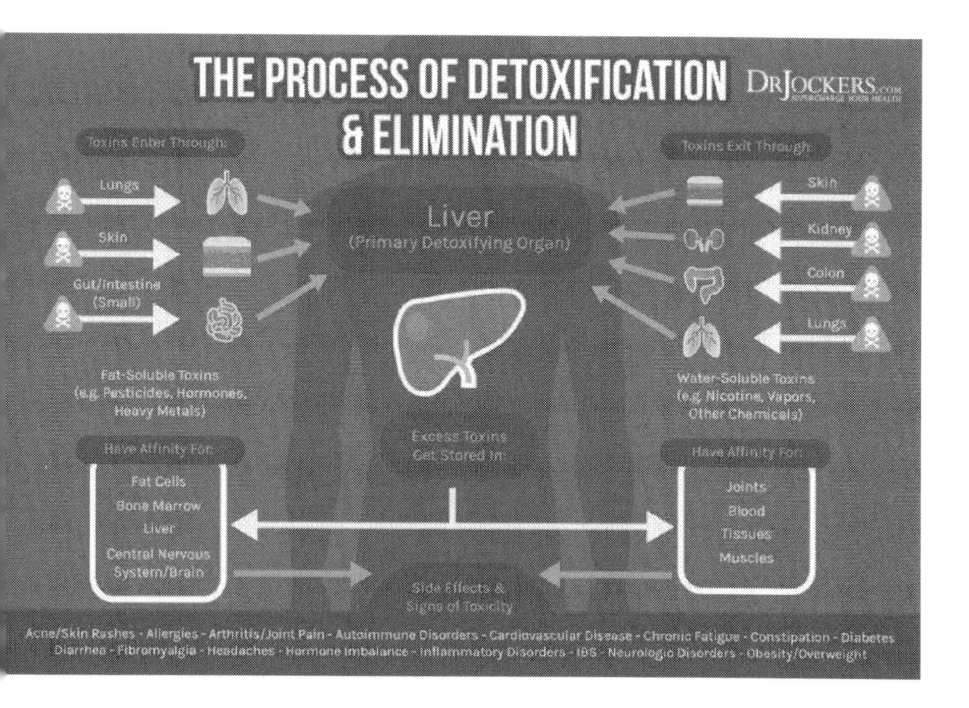

Challenge #4: Re-feeding Syndrome

Re-feeding syndrome is a very rare, yet quite dangerous, complication that can occur from extended fasting or chronic malnourishment. Upon re-feeding, intracellular and blood electrolyte levels experience a temporary shift.

While most people can handle this shift with no problems, it is still important to understand how to minimize your risk.

Re-feeding syndrome occurs mostly in people who are severely deficient in phosphorus. Because phosphorus is prevalent in most foods, people who are mostly at risk are those with eating disorders or other conditions which have created chronic malnourishment such as anorexia or alcoholism.

Other factors that are important to note in determining the risk of this dangerous electrolyte shift are:

- Salt intake during the fast
- The intensity of insulin stimulation following the fast (how hard you spike your blood sugar upon re-feeding)

This is why I recommend electrolyte intake while fasting and a gradual introduction of low-glycemic foods upon breaking the fast. Following these recommendations will make this already rare phenomenon a non-issue.

Challenge #5: Feeling Cold

Once you reach the 18–24-hour mark of a fast, you may start to experience cold hands, feet, or all over. This phenomenon affects different people at different intensities. While some people may experience a very mild chill on the fingers, others may feel the need to layer on sweatshirts or turn on the heat.

While this can be uncomfortable or concerning for some people, it is actually a sign that fasting is doing beneficial things in your body.

Research shows that fasting stimulates the parasympathetic nervous system (1). Stimulation of the parasympathetic nervous system promotes a state of relaxation which also reduces blood pressure, heart rate, and body temperature (2).

This is a completely normal adaptation to fasting. The body is trying to conserve energy that it would normally use to produce heat and is diverting that energy towards healing and repair.

Getting a bit of light exercise, taking a warm bath, sitting in the sauna, making sure you are getting enough salt, and layering up can all help you get through this beneficial change.

With time, feelings of coldness should decrease as your body becomes better adapted to fasting.

Supplements to Support Fasting

Taking certain types of supplements during a fast can be extremely beneficial if:

- You want to eliminate or drastically reduce fasting side effects
- You want to get maximum benefits out of your fast
- You have particular health benefits you are targeting

While our ancestors didn't necessarily take supplements when they fasted, I do believe that we can take advantage of particular benefits by using them in specific ways. Ultimately, how healing a particular strategy is for you is determined by how well you are able to adhere to it. Using particular supplements can make the fasting experience more comfortable and increase your success.

This can be especially helpful in the beginning stages of fasting as those initial successes in your health endeavors will build confidence and momentum towards future efforts.

Will Taking Supplements Break a Fast?

I get asked this all the time and here's what I have to say about it... sometimes, and technically yes – but not really. I know, that's really confusing but it's actually easy to understand with a little bit of understanding of how certain supplements affect insulin levels.

Many fasting purists will say absolutely, without a doubt, supplements will break your fast. Technically, you are consuming something solid. The nuance to this is that, if that supplement does not stimulate insulin levels, then it will not negatively impact things like fat-burning, ketosis, or growth hormone.

This is my stance on fasting supplementation. If it does not stimulate an insulin response, then it is most likely fine.

If your supplement contains any amount of glucose or sugar, especially in excess of 20 calories, then chances are that it will create an insulinogenic response. Although very minimal, if you are looking for maximum benefits then you'd want to avoid those supplements.

Other supplements you would want to avoid while fasting are those that are designated to be taken with food. These are things like zinc, iron, multi-vitamins, oil supplements (fish, hemp, etc.), and digestive supplements such as betaine HCL and digestive enzymes.

Reasons to Supplement While Fasting

In my years of experience there are 5 major scenarios in which taking supplements while fasting can be helpful:

1. Dehydration and Electrolyte Depletion
2. Hypoglycemia
3. Excessive Oxidative Stress
4. Gut Induced Endotoxemia
5. Fat Cell Induced Endotoxemia

I want to briefly touch on each of these scenarios, how they can cause fasting challenges, and what supplements I recommend to combat them. First, let's discuss dehydration.

1. Dehydration and Electrolyte Depletion

This will be brief because I think I've really hammered this one in over the course of this book. When you fast, for a number of reasons, your body will quickly deplete water and electrolyte levels.

Dehydration and/or electrolyte depletion will lead to a wide range of potential symptoms such as:

- Changes in heartrate
- Muscle spasms and cramps
- Anxiety and sleep problems
- Dizziness
- Fatigue
- Headaches
- Low blood pressure

While many of these symptoms can also occur for things like hypoglycemia and endotoxemia (both of which we will discuss shortly) staying hydrated is step one in optimizing your body for fasting.

Supplements for Supporting Hydration

Electrolytes: Help your body retain water by upping your electrolyte intake. Make the fasting solution I've discussed previously in this book or find a capsulated electrolyte formula that is free from calories.

Ketone Salts: Another great option to support hydration and ketosis for a smooth transition into fasting is a ketone salt formula. Ketone salts are ketones (what your body turns fat into for energy) bound to electrolytes like sodium, magnesium, and potassium. While they don't taste the best, they can be great for mitigating many fasting side effects by improving hydration and ketone levels simultaneously.

2. Hypoglycemia

Hypoglycemic responses are normal during fasting. The intensity of which you experience hypoglycemia will depend on your mitochondrial health and how much you've metabolically prepared your body for fasting previously.

That being said, at least mild and temporary hypoglycemic responses should be expected for most fasters.

Temporary hypoglycemia when there are not adequate ketone levels in the blood will create an energy deficit in the brain which can lead to symptoms such as:

- Dizziness
- Fatigue
- Brain fog
- Headaches
- Mood changes
- Anxiety
- Food cravings
- Insomnia

You will notice that the symptoms of hypoglycemia are almost exactly the same as those of dehydration. This is likely because insulin changes and hydration levels are linked in many ways.

Consequently, I would approach alleviation of hypoglycemic symptoms very similarly to dehydration. First address hydration levels, then consider the supplements below.

Supplements for Supporting Hypoglycemia

Magnesium: As one of the most abundant and diversely used minerals in the body, low magnesium levels cause a lot of problems. When the body is under higher amounts of stress, such is the case while fasting, magnesium is used up at an accelerated rate. Interestingly enough, magnesium deficiency symptoms are almost identical to low blood sugar symptoms.

Increasing magnesium intake through the use of a ketone salt or a chelated magnesium supplement is very helpful while fasting. Not all forms are absorbed effectively though. Good forms to use would include:

- Magnesium malate
- Magnesium citrate
- Magnesium glycinate
- Magnesium orotate
- Magnesium taurate
- Magnesium L-threonate (especially good for crossing into the brain to calm stress)

Adaptogenic Herbs: Low blood sugar is a stressful event for the body and can lead to an elevation in cortisol. This is a natural response as cortisol helps to retrieve stored carbohydrate from the liver and muscle cells to keep blood sugar stable.

If you are someone who is healing from poor health, chances are your body either over or under-produces cortisol and does not regulate blood sugar efficiently.

An adaptogen is a compound that helps the body deal with this cortisol response more efficiently. By doing so we can assist the body in restoring a normal blood sugar balance and experience less symptoms.

Some of the most well-studied adaptogens include:

- Ashwagandha
- Rhodiola
- Holy basil
- Ginseng
- Cordyceps
- Reishi mushroom
- Lion's mane

There are plenty of options available for adaptogens on the market. For best results make sure you look for organic or wild-crafted adaptogens with 3rd party testing for heavy metals, pesticides, and other common toxins. Finding an adaptogenic herb blend can be powerful as well. Make sure to find a product that is free from calories!

Exogenous Ketones: I've already discussed exogenous ketones for assistance in hydration, but they are also great for beating hypoglycemia symptoms. Low blood sugar in the absence of adequate ketone levels is an issue. If the body has adequate ketone levels, however, then it is unlikely that you will feel any symptoms of hypoglycemia. This is if your body is adapted to burning them.

Especially if you are newer to fasting, your body has to become accustomed to having elevated ketones in the blood to adapt to using them as energy. By providing ketones from an exogenous source, we speed up this process and provide the brain with energy.

3. Excessive Oxidative Stress

Oxidative stress is a good thing. In fact, even inflammation is good when it occurs in the right amounts. When oxidative stress becomes out of control, then we get problems. Because fasting is a stressor and many tissues are going through rapid changes, oxidative stress may increase. A large part of this increase in oxidative stress may be from toxicity release which we will discuss next.

Oxidative stress is increased by compounds called free radicals. Free radicals are otherwise harmless compounds that have lost an electron and become unstable. In order to re-stabilize themselves, free radicals must steal electrons from around the body. Oftentimes these electrons come from the mitochondria or cell membranes. This results in damaged cells and inhibited energy production.

Chances are, if you have excess body fat, a history of gut issues, or are battling serious health challenges – you will face large amounts of oxidative stress as your body heals itself.

Supplement Support for Oxidative Stress

Hydrogen: Hydrogen is the smallest atomic gas molecule that acts as an anti-oxidant by donating an electron to free radicals. This helps to stabilize them and make them unable to damage other healthy cells.

Hydrogen is so small that it is able to penetrate down to the cellular level. Another great thing about hydrogen is that it selectively quenches the most harmful free radicals while allowing beneficial oxidative stress processes to continue.

There is a great deal of research on hydrogen and it has been found to:

- Relieve oxidative stress with no side effects (3)
- Protects against cellular damage (4)
- Protects against mitochondrial damage (5)
- Protects against DNA damage

Hydrogen-rich water is one of the supplements I highly advocate for anyone during a fast. You can buy hydrogen-rich water or make your own with hydrogen water by using molecular hydrogen tablets that you simply dissolve in a glass of water.

4. Gut induced Endotoxemia

As we've discussed several times so far, the gut microbiome changes drastically during extended fasting.

Your microbiome is made up of trillions of microorganisms like bacteria, yeast, amoeba, viruses, and sometimes parasites. When the microbiome is in good balance it defends you against toxins and unwanted microbes while also creating nutrients your body needs.

When the microbiome is not in good balance, unwanted microbes can create toxins and steal nutrients from your body – creating a source of chronic inflammation (4). This is what most people who follow a standard American diet or have a history of antibiotic use deal with.

When fasting, these harmful microbes quickly die off. While this is a good thing long-term, this can create acute toxicity and inflammation in the body. This can sometimes manifest as skin rashes, headaches, increased body odor, brain fog, and fatigue.
Another reason that toxicity can stem from the gut is if you have stool trapped in your gut that has not been moved in several days. This is why supporting your body to clear your bowels within the first two days of an extended fast is really important. I notice a drastic difference in how I feel at days 3–5 when I have had thorough bowel movements in the beginning stages of my fast.

With the above considered, the best supplements to support you will be those that assist in bowel movements and bind to biotoxins such as those released from bacterial die-off.

Supplements to Support a Healthy Gut Environment While Fasting

Activated Charcoal, Bioactive Carbon, or other binders: The first step in preventing unwanted effects of gut-mediated endotoxemia is to prevent the opportunity for endotoxin to enter the blood stream. The best way to do this is to consume a compound that has a high binding-ability within the gut. Taking things like activated charcoal, bioactive carbon, or bentonite clay.

Bioactive carbons, as I've mentioned, are a relatively newer compound that have the ability to pass through the gut and even help bind toxins within the blood stream. In my opinion, this capability makes bioactive carbons my preferred binder over charcoal and clay, but they do cost more as well. Activated charcoal is the lowest cost binder and it works most specifically in the gut.

Oxygen-based Intestinal Cleanser: Using a gentle intestinal cleanser is powerful at the beginning of a fast. Simply put, if you don't clear your bowels before a fast, chances are it's going to sit in there... and for the reasons above – you don't want that.

I would highly suggest using an oxygen-based intestinal cleanser such as OxyPowder, receiving a colonic, or doing a coffee enema during the first full day of fasting to reduce the impact of endotoxins and optimize the benefits of your fast.

5. **Fat Cell induced Endotoxemia**

One of the double-edged swords of fasting is that:

1. It is excellent for quickly burning excess fat off the body to maintain a healthy metabolism

   BUT

2. Fat also happens to be where our bodies store a lot of the toxins we encounter on a daily basis

So yes, while you are restoring a healthy body weight (which has innumerous health benefits) you may also experience a temporary reaction from the body as stored toxins are released from your fat cells.

If you are a healthy person, you would be constantly eliminating toxins through respiration, perspiration, urination, and defecation.

Unfortunately, many people have unintentionally exposed themselves to so much toxicity that they have compromised these detoxification systems.

If you already have backed-up detoxification systems, then once those toxins become released from your fat stores it might cause some issues. If drainage pathways are moving slowly, then these fat-cell derived endotoxins will accumulate and elicit a strong inflammatory response.

This is another reason to make sure you move your bowels well at the beginning of a fast and continue to drink enough water throughout to maintain efficient detoxification.

Supplements to Support Detoxification Systems and Inflammation

Bioactive Carbon: In this scenario, some type of bioactive carbon (fulvic and humic acids) are going to be your best bet. As I stated in the previous section, bioactive carbons are able to pass through the intestinal tract and bind to toxins in the blood stream. This is something that activated charcoals or bentonite clay cannot do.

Hydrogen-Rich Water: In addition to binding the toxins quickly, you would also want to mitigate any inflammation as efficiently as possible to avoid the side effects. Hydrogen-rich water is by far one of the best ways to reduce inflammation quickly.

Top Supplements for Fasting Recap

- **Electrolytes** – Aids hydration, prevents weakness, dizziness, headaches
- **Ketone Salts –** Aids hydration, assists with cravings, provides energy
- **Magnesium –** Aids blood sugar, prevents symptoms of hypoglycemia, calms the mind
- **Adaptogenic Herbs –** Reduces cortisol, levels blood sugar, improves sleep
- **Hydrogen –** Calms inflammation, provides mental clarity, assists overall healing
- **Activated Charcoal or Bentonite Clay –** Bind toxins within the digestive tract
- **Bioactive Carbons** – Bind toxins within the digestive tract and within the blood stream
- **Oxygen-Based Intestinal Cleanser** – Assists with clearing the bowels to prevent gut-mediated endotoxemia

Chapter 12: The Fasting Lifestyle

We've learned a lot about fasting in this book. While fasting is an effective health strategy for many reasons, it is ultimately another tool in your toolbelt used to achieve the best life possible.

If there is anything that my time in Functional Medicine has taught me, it's that nothing works for everyone the same way. Some people will do great on a ketogenic diet, some a carnivore diet, and some a Mediterranean diet. Some people need extended fasting and others will do much better with a daily 12–14 hour fast.

While there is not a single solution for everyone, there is some variation of fasting that can fit into your lifestyle.

It all begins with trying it out and slowly dialing in what your body needs over time.

So Let's Recap...

Fasting has been a part of human life since we have existed. While this may have initially developed as a survival mechanism for times of food scarcity, current research has shown fasting to be a powerful tool to fight the diseases of modern excess.

Namely, cancer, diabetes, obesity, and heart disease... Basically everything that happens to us when we eat poorly and don't exercise enough.

In the beginning of this book we discussed how there is a huge societal dogma that says fasting and starving yourself are the same thing. This would suggest that fasting is an unhealthy behavior that we should be avoiding.

Well, I think at this point we've uncovered enough evidence to show that this is absolutely not the case! Fasting is powerful and desperately needed by people in our society.

We don't need to spend billions of dollars every year on surgeries and medications when we have such a powerful and free tool at our disposal. We just need more people who understand how to use it properly.

The Most Important Benefits of Fasting That We've Uncovered Include:

Healing a broken metabolism and burning body fat

A poor ability to burn body fat is likely the number one contributing factor to chronic disease and all-cause mortality. When your body becomes poor at regulating energy, a lot of things go wrong.

Fasting is the quickest way to restore your body's ability to burn fat and begin reversing this risk.

Quickly restoring insulin sensitivity

When the metabolism goes awry, insulin resistance is almost always a factor. When you overfill your body with sugar, it begins to not let any more in.

This make your brain think that your starving even though you are more than well-fed. Then you get stuck in the cycle of eating yet never feeling truly satiated or energized. Fasting is the fastest way to deplete the excess sugar and restore insulin sensitivity.

Reducing inflammation

Chronic inflammatory conditions such as autoimmunity, skin disorders, digestive issues, and even depression are rampant. These conditions often develop from the gut.

If you don't have a healthy gut, chances are you are moving your body towards one of the listed conditions. Fasting allows the digestive system to heal and reset itself by allowing it to rest.

Keeping cells young by promoting autophagy and upregulating stem cell production

Sometimes cells get old and they hang around for too long. This prevents the development of new healthy cells.

Fasting helps take care of this by quickly targeting the old cells and stimulating stem cells to rejuvenate damaged tissue. The result is rapid healing!

Promoting youthful hormone balance by keeping insulin levels in check

Insulin is an anti-youth hormone. You simply cannot have elevated insulin and growth hormone at the same time. In fact, the lower your insulin is, the higher your growth hormone tends to be! Fasting lowers insulin quite effectively and consequently this does a lot of amazing things for the hormones that keep you young and feeling energized.

Reducing the risk of every chronic disease related to the metabolism

Metabolic diseases are the biggest killer of humans worldwide. Things like heart disease, cancer, dementia, diabetes, and depression can all be related back to having a disrupted metabolism. Fasting may be the most effective and affordable answer for this problem.

Improving your relationship with food so that it no longer takes control of your day

Most of us grew up eating 3 meals a day plus snacks... That's a lot of time during the day to be consumed by the planning, preparation, and consumption of food! Additionally, many people fall back on food as a drug to cope with boredom. Fasting relieves you of this stimulus and allows you to evaluate your relationship with food.

Improving mental health and focus

Chronic inflammation and poor blood sugar control are both implicated in a wide variety of mental ailments from depression to dementia. Fasting improves blood sugar control while promoting the formation of ketones. Many people find that running on ketones as a primary fuel source provides a sense of calm and mental clarity that they have not experienced with any other health strategy.

Boosting energy levels through mitochondrial biogenesis

By promoting ketosis and stimulating the growth of new mitochondria, fasting is kind of like its own form of exercise. Doing it regularly keeps your mitochondria healthy and ensures you have plenty of energy for your daily tasks.

Healing the digestive system

Digestive issues are a big red flag that can create chronic inflammation. Ultimately, chronic digestive issues can lead to many things that you don't want. Fasting is great way to give your digestion a break and quickly heal the gut lining.

Providing clarity in matters of intuition, spiritual guidance, and decision making

We have so many distractions affecting us on a daily basis. This interferes with our ability to focus and gain clarity on things that are important to us. This is likely why so many cultures and religions have partaken in fasting for thousands of years to deepen their connections with the source of their inspiration. Fasting clears the mind and provides a unique edge of focus that allows us to gain clarity in important decisions.

Creating the Fasting Schedule That Fits your Needs

By now you should understand that there is no optimal fasting schedule that works for everyone. In fact, the fasting schedule that you thrive on may cause issues for someone else.

This is why it is so important to experiment and figure out what works for you.

The most efficient way I can recommend for finding your ideal fasting schedule is to follow the recommended implementation in Chapter 8. Start with a daily 12-hour fast, then slowly work your way up to an extended water fast.

By the time you have progressed through the fasting levels, you will have a good understanding of what works well for your schedule while also making you feel amazing.

For example, I tend to wake up early and complete my most mentally demanding work first thing in the morning. I feel the most mentally sharp when I am fasting so I almost always fast at least 16 hours per day.

In addition to this, I have found that I respond well to fairly regular 24-hour fasts. My current fasting schedule consists of daily 16–18 hour fasts along with 2, 20–24-hour fasts spaced several days apart.

This fasting schedule merges very well with my work schedule and allows me to stay very productive while staying healthy.

Here is a quick recap of the schedule from Chapter 8:

Week 1 & Week 2: Eliminate sugar with a daily 12–14 hour fast
Week 3: Crescendo or cycle fasting with ketogenic refeeds
Week 4: Daily 16–18 hour fast with ketogenic refeeds
Week 5: Add a 24-hour fat fast, once per week
Week 6: Add a 24-hour water fast, once or twice per week

Once a 24-hour fast can be completed comfortably, you are ready to attempt 3–5 days of partial or water fasting.

Use the fasting strength questionnaire to determine if you are adapting well to your current fasting schedule and if you are ready for the next step! If you aren't adapting well, it is ok, follow the instructions on how to reset your stress response and gradually build up your fasting fitness level.

Benefits of Feast-Famine Cycling

DrJockers.com

- Regulates Cell Growth and Cleansing Pathways
- Creates Hormonal Optimization
- Improves Lean Body Tissue Development
- Stimulates Fat Burning
- Balances Inflammation and Immune Activity
- Enhances Mental and Emotional Well-Being

****Going through phases of feasting on nutrient dense foods and periods of intermittent and extended fasting improves our metabolic flexibility and energy efficiency and makes us incredibly strong and resilient human beings.*

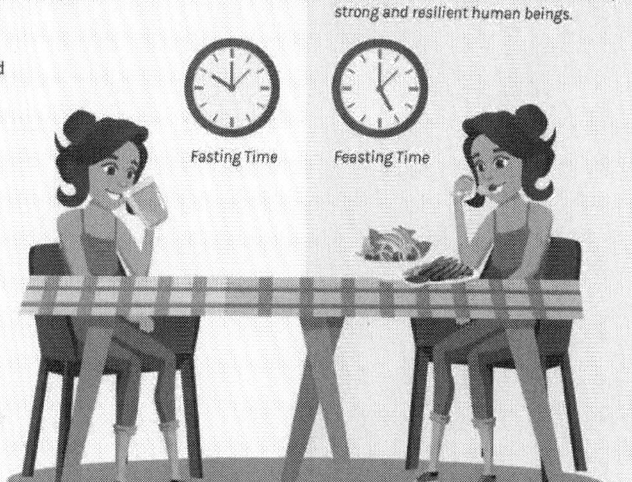

TIMES OF FEASTING
Growth, Building and Reproduction is Favored over Cell Cleansing and Healing

TIMES OF FASTING
Cell Cleansing and Healing is Favored over Growth, Building and Reproduction

Importance of Feast-Famine Cycling

Prolonged periods of caloric restriction wreak havoc on your metabolism. This is why traditional diets don't usually work very well. The longer you go without adequate calories, the slower your metabolism becomes.

Feast-famine cycling fixes this flaw by only allowing the body to go through brief periods of caloric restriction followed by periods of caloric surplus.

For those who are obese or overweight, this cycle ensures weight loss occurs at a steadier rate with less chance of plateau.

Feast-famine cycling is even more important for people who are lean and do not have excess body fat. Those who are lean are extra sensitive to caloric deficits and can quickly have thyroid, stress and sex hormone disruptions if intermittent periods of caloric surplus are not also present.

If you are a lean individual looking for a performance boost while optimizing lean body mass, then you would want to stick to daily fasting strategies while ensuring adequate calories are consumed during feeding windows.

My personal fasting routine works excellent with my workout schedule as it keeps my energy levels high, keeps me lean, and I never worry about losing muscle mass.

My coauthor Michael has adopted a unique approach where he will follow an OMAD schedule on some days while eating breakfast and dinner on other days. He ensures to schedule breakfast and dinner in a way that allows for a minimum of 10 hours of no eating between meals. On this schedule, Michael was able to put on 24lbs of muscle in a 3-month period with zero fat gain.

Michael and I both also partake in fairly regular multi-day water fasts.

While I have adopted a mix of fasting styles, you may find that daily 14-hour fasts work great for you. You may also find that all you need is an occasional 72-hour fast! That's the beauty of fasting, most styles of fasting have benefits and can be molded to your preferences.

Thank You

If you've made it through this entire book, I hope you are ready to take action on the wealth of knowledge inside. I hope you have found it transformative and empowering on your path to optimal health.

Whether you are someone battling disease or you are looking for an edge in your daily performance, I believe fasting can be a powerful tool for you.

I want to say thank you for investing your valuable time and trusting me with your health.

This book has been a career in the making as I continue to learn from the research that has been conducted and the thousands of patients that have come through my clinic.

Thank you for reading and I wish you all the best on your journey towards optimal living!

References

Chapter 1

1 Saklayen MG. The Global Epidemic of the Metabolic Syndrome. Curr Hypertens Rep. 2018;20(2):12.

2 Patterson, R. E., Laughlin, G. A., LaCroix, A. Z., Hartman, S. J., Natarajan, L., Senger, C. M., Martínez, M. E., Villaseñor, A., Sears, D. D., Marinac, C. R., ... Gallo, L. C. Intermittent Fasting and Human Metabolic Health. *Journal of the Academy of Nutrition and Dietetics*. 2005. *115*(8), 1203-12. PMCID: 4516560

3 Knight, W. D., Witte, M. M., Parsons, A. D., Gierach, M., & Overton, J. M. Long-term caloric restriction reduces metabolic rate and heart rate under cool and thermoneutral conditions in FBNF1 rats. *Mechanisms of ageing and development*. 2011.*132*(5), 220-9. PMCID: 3118456

4 Moller L, et al. Impact of fasting on growth hormone signaling and action in muscle and fat. 2009 Mar. *J Clin Endocrinol Metab*. 94(3): 965-72. PMID: 19066303

5 Johnstone, A. Fasting for weight loss: an effective strategy or latest diet trend? *Int J Obes (Lond)*. 2015 May. 39(5): 727-33. PMID: 25540982

6 Patterson RE, Laughlin GA, LaCroix AZ, et al. Intermittent Fasting and Human Metabolic Health. *J Acad Nutr Diet*. 2015; 115(8):1203-12. PMCID: 4516560

7 Faris MA, et al. "Intermittent Fasting During Ramadan Attenuates Pro-inflammatory Cytokines and Immune Cells in Healthy Subjects.." *Nutrition Research*, Vol. 32, No. 12, Dec 2012.

8 Mohan, ML et al. "Proinflammatory Cytokines Mediate GPCR Dysfunction" Journal of cardiovascular pharmacology Vol. 70, No. 2, Aug 2017.

9 Zhang, Jun-Ming and An, Jianxiong. "Cytokines, Inflammation, and Pain" *International Anesthesiology Clinics*, Vol. 45, No. 2, Spring 2007.

10 Spranger J, et al. "Inflammatory Cytokines and the Risk to Develop Type 2 Diabetes: Results of the Prospective Population-Based European Prospective Investigation into Cancer and Nutrition (EPIC)-Potsdam Study." *Diabetes*, Vol. 52, No. 3, Mar 2003.

11 Fann, DY, et al. Intermittent fasting attenuates inflammasome activity in ischemic stroke. *Exp Neurol*. 2014 Jul. 257:114-9. PMID: 24805069

12 Alirezaei M, Kemball CC, Flynn CT, Wood MR, Whitton JL, Kiosses WB. Short-term fasting induces profound neuronal autophagy. Autophagy. 2010;6(6):702-10.

13 Longo VD, Mattson MP. Fasting: molecular mechanisms and clinical applications. Cell Metab. 2014;19(2):181-92.

14 Cheng CW, Adams GB, Perin L, et al. Prolonged fasting reduces IGF-1/PKA to promote hematopoietic-stem-cell-based regeneration and reverse immunosuppression. *Cell Stem Cell*. 2014; 14(6):810-23. PMCID: 4102383

15 Mendelsohn AR, and Larrick JW. Prolonged fasting/refeeding promotes hematopoietic stem cell regeneration and rejuvenation. *Rejuvenation Res*. 2014 Aug. 17(4): 385-9. PMID: 25072352

16 Intermountain Healthcare: New Research Finds Routine Periodic Fasting is Good for Your Health, and Your Heart Link Here

17 Saklayen MG. The Global Epidemic of the Metabolic Syndrome. Curr Hypertens Rep. 2018;20(2):12.

18 Mattson MP, Longo VD, Harvie M. Impact of intermittent fasting on health and disease processes. *Ageing Res Rev*. 2016; 39:46-58. PMCID: 5411330

19 Fond G, Macgregor A, Leboyer M, and Michalsen A. Fasting in mood disorders: neurobiology and effectiveness. A review of the literature. *Psychiatry Res*. 2013 Oct. 209 (3): 253-8. PMID: 23332541

20 Mihaylova MM, et al. Fasting Activates Fatty Acid Oxidation to Enhance Intestinal Stem Cell Function during Homeostasis and Aging. *Cell Stem Cell*. 2018 May. 22(5): 769-778. PMID: 29727683

Chapter 2

1 Insulin resistance and prediabetes. National Institute of Diabetes and Digestive and Kidney Diseases. Link Here

2 López-otín C, Galluzzi L, Freije JMP, Madeo F, Kroemer G. Metabolic Control of Longevity. Cell. 2016;166(4):802-821.

3 Diabetes. Mayo Clinic. Link Here
4 Blood Sugar Test. Medline Plus. Link Here
5 Diagnosing diabetes and learning about prediabetes. American Diabetes Association. Link Here
6 Belkacemi L, Selselet-attou G, Louchami K, Sener A, Malaisse WJ. Intermittent fasting modulation of the diabetic syndrome in sand rats. II. In vivo investigations. Int J Mol Med. 2010;26(5):759-65.
7 Hatori M, Vollmers C, Zarrinpar A, et al. Time-restricted feeding without reducing caloric intake prevents metabolic diseases in mice fed a high-fat diet. Cell Metab. 2012;15(6):848-60.
8 Godar RJ, Ma X, Liu H, et al. Repetitive stimulation of autophagy-lysosome machinery by intermittent fasting preconditions the myocardium to ischemia-reperfusion injury. Autophagy. 2015;11(9):1537-60.
9 Katare RG, Kakinuma Y, Arikawa M, Yamasaki F, Sato T. Chronic intermittent fasting improves the survival following large myocardial ischemia by activation of BDNF/VEGF/PI3K signaling pathway. J Mol Cell Cardiol. 2009;46(3):405-12.
10 Castello L, Froio T, Maina M, et al. Alternate-day fasting protects the rat heart against age-induced inflammation and fibrosis by inhibiting oxidative damage and NF-kB activation. Free Radic Biol Med. 2010;48(1):47-54.
11 Wan R, Camandola S, Mattson MP. Intermittent food deprivation improves cardiovascular and neuroendocrine responses to stress in rats. J Nutr. 2003;133(6):1921-9.
12 Varady KA, Roohk DJ, Loe YC, Mcevoy-hein BK, Hellerstein MK. Effects of modified alternate-day fasting regimens on adipocyte size, triglyceride metabolism, and plasma adiponectin levels in mice. J Lipid Res. 2007;48(10):2212-9.
13 Belkacemi L, Selselet-attou G, Hupkens E, et al. Intermittent fasting modulation of the diabetic syndrome in streptozotocin-injected rats. Int J Endocrinol. 2012;2012:962012.
14 Chaix A, Zarrinpar A, Miu P, Panda S. Time-restricted feeding is a preventative and therapeutic intervention against diverse nutritional challenges. Cell Metab. 2014;20(6):991-1005.
15 Arumugam TV, Phillips TM, Cheng A, Morrell CH, Mattson MP, Wan R. Age and energy intake interact to modify cell stress pathways and stroke outcome. Ann Neurol. 2010;67(1):41-52.
16 Lee C, Longo VD. Fasting vs dietary restriction in cellular protection and cancer treatment: from model organisms to patients. Oncogene. 2011;30(30):3305-16.
17 Tinsley GM, La bounty PM. Effects of intermittent fasting on body composition and clinical health markers in humans. Nutr Rev. 2015;73(10):661-74.
18 Seimon RV, Roekenes JA, Zibellini J, et al. Do intermittent diets provide physiological benefits over continuous diets for weight loss? A systematic review of clinical trials. Mol Cell Endocrinol. 2015;418 Pt 2:153-72.
19 Mattson MP, Longo VD, Harvie M. Impact of intermittent fasting on health and disease processes. Ageing Res Rev. 2017;39:46-58.
20 Steckhan, N., Hohmann, C.-D., Kessler, C., Dobos, G., Michalsen, A., & Cramer, H. (2016). Effects of different dietary approaches on inflammatory markers in patients with metabolic syndrome: A systematic review and meta-analysis. *Nutrition*, *32*(3), 338–348. PMID: 26706026
21 Raygan, F., Bahmani, F., Kouchaki, E., Aghadavod, E., Sharifi, S., Akbari, E., . . . Asemi, Z. (2016). Comparative effects of carbohydrate versus fat restriction on metabolic profiles, biomarkers of inflammation and oxidative stress 5. in overweight patients with Type 2 diabetic and coronary heart disease: A randomized clinical trial. PMID: 28607566
22 Gershuni VM, Yan SL, Medici V. Nutritional Ketosis for Weight Management and Reversal of Metabolic Syndrome. Curr Nutr Rep. 2018;7(3):97-106.
23 Mattson MP, Moehl K, Ghena N, Schmaedick M, Cheng A. Intermittent metabolic switching, neuroplasticity and brain health. Nat Rev Neurosci. 2018;19(2):63-80.
24 Kimura I, Inoue D, Maeda T, et al. Short-chain fatty acids and ketones directly regulate sympathetic nervous system via G protein-coupled receptor 41 (GPR41). Proc Natl Acad Sci USA. 2011;108(19):8030-5.
25 Wilhelmi de toledo F, Grundler F, Bergouignan A, Drinda S, Michalsen A. Safety, health improvement and well-being during a 4 to 21-day fasting period in an observational study including 1422 subjects. PLoS ONE. 2019;14(1):e0209353.
26 Lu J, Tan M, Cai Q. The Warburg effect in tumor progression: mitochondrial oxidative metabolism as an anti-metastasis mechanism. Cancer Lett. 2015;356(2 Pt A):156-64.

27 Seyfried TN, Yu G, Maroon JC, D'agostino DP. Press-pulse: a novel therapeutic strategy for the metabolic management of cancer. Nutr Metab (Lond). 2017;14:19.
28 Seyfried TN, Mukherjee P, Iyikesici MS, et al. Consideration of Ketogenic Metabolic Therapy as a Complementary or Alternative Approach for Managing Breast Cancer. Front Nutr. 2020;7:21.
29 Seyfried TN, Shelton L, Arismendi-morillo G, et al. Provocative Question: Should Ketogenic Metabolic Therapy Become the Standard of Care for Glioblastoma?. Neurochem Res. 2019;44(10):2392-2404.
30 Dąbek A, Wojtala M, Pirola L, Balcerczyk A. Modulation of Cellular Biochemistry, Epigenetics and Metabolomics by Ketone Bodies. Implications of the Ketogenic Diet in the Physiology of the Organism and Pathological States. Nutrients. 2020;12(3)
31 Miller VJ, Villamena FA, Volek JS. Nutritional Ketosis and Mitohormesis: Potential Implications for Mitochondrial Function and Human Health. J Nutr Metab. 2018;2018:5157645.
32 Masternak MM, Bartke A. Growth hormone, inflammation and aging. *Pathobiology of Aging & Age Related Diseases*. 2012;2:10.3402/pba.v2i0.17293. doi:10.3402/pba.v2i0.17293.
33 Rudman D, Feller AG, Nagraj HS, et al. Effects of human growth hormone in men over 60 years old. N Engl J Med. 1990;323(1):1-6.
34 Blackman MR, Sorkin JD, Münzer T, et al. Growth hormone and sex steroid administration in healthy aged women and men: a randomized controlled trial. JAMA. 2002;288(18):2282-92.
35 Ho KY, Veldhuis JD, Johnson ML, Furlanetto R, Evans WS, Alberti KG, Thorner MO. Fasting enhances growth hormone secretion and amplifies the complex rhythms of growth hormone secretion in man. J Clin Invest. 1988 Apr;81(4):968-75. PMID: 312742
36 Vendelbo MH, Jørgensen JO, Pedersen SB, Gormsen LC, Lund S, Schmitz O, Jessen N, Møller N. Exercise and fasting activate growth hormone-dependent myocellular signal transducer and activator of transcription-5b phosphorylation and insulin-like growth factor-I messenger ribonucleic acid expression in humans. J Clin Endocrinol Metab. 2010 Sep;95(9):E64-8. PMID:20534752
37 Yamamoto M, Iguchi G, Fukuoka H, Suda K, Bando H, Takahashi M, Nishizawa H, Seino S, Takahashi Y. SIRT1 regulates adaptive response of the growth hormone–insulin-like growth factor-I axis under fasting conditions in liver. Proc Natl Acad Sci U S A. 2013 Sep 10;110(37):14948-53. PMID:23980167
38 Farzad Hayati, Mohsen Maleki, Maryam Pourmohammad, Kamran Sardari, Mehrdad Mohri, Amir Afkhami. Influence of Short-term, Repeated Fasting on the Skin Wound Healing of Female Mice. Woundsresearch.com. Link Here
39 Hartman ML, Veldhuis JD, Johnson ML, et al. Augmented growth hormone (GH) secretory burst frequency and amplitude mediate enhanced GH secretion during a two-day fast in normal men. J Clin Endocrinol Metab. 1992;74(4):757-65.
40 Westbrook R, Bonkowski MS, Arum O, Strader AD, Bartke A. Metabolic alterations due to caloric restriction and every other day feeding in normal and growth hormone receptor knockout mice. J Gerontol A Biol Sci Med Sci. 2014;69(1):25-33.
41 Salminen A, Kaarniranta K. AMP-activated protein kinase (AMPK) controls the aging process via an integrated signaling network. Ageing Res Rev. 2012;11(2):230-41.
42 Wijngaarden, M. A., van der Zon, G. C., van Dijk, K. W., Pijl, H., & Guigas, B. (2013). Effects of prolonged fasting on AMPK signaling, gene expression, and mitochondrial respiratory chain content in skeletal muscle from lean and obese individuals. *American Journal of Physiology-Endocrinology and Metabolism*, *304*(9), E1012-E1021.
43 Bujak AL, Crane JD, Lally JS, et al. AMPK activation of muscle autophagy prevents fasting-induced hypoglycemia and myopathy during aging. Cell Metab. 2015;21(6):883-90.
44 Reya T, Morrison SJ, Clarke MF, Weissman IL. Stem cells, cancer, and cancer stem cells. Nature. 2001;414:105–11.
45 Adams PD, Jasper H, Rudolph KL. Aging-Induced Stem Cell Mutations as Drivers for Disease and Cancer. Cell Stem Cell. 2015;16:601–12.
46 Brandhorst S, Choi IY, Wei M, et al. A Periodic Diet that Mimics Fasting Promotes Multi-System Regeneration, Enhanced Cognitive Performance, and Healthspan. Cell Metab. 2015;22(1):86-99.
47 Mana MD, Kuo EY, Yilmaz ÖH. Dietary Regulation of Adult Stem Cells. Curr Stem Cell Rep. 2017;3(1):1-8.

Chapter 3

1 Varady KA, Bhutani S, Church EC, Klempel MC. Short-term modified alternate-day fasting: a novel dietary strategy for weight loss and cardioprotection in obese adults. Am J Clin Nutr. 2009;90(5):1138-43. PMID: 19793855

2 Arnason TG, Bowen MW, Mansell KD. Effects of intermittent fasting on health markers in those with type 2 diabetes: A pilot study. World J Diabetes. 2017;8(4):154-164. PMID: 28465792

3 Muñoz-hernández L, Márquez-lópez Z, Mehta R, Aguilar-salinas CA. Intermittent Fasting as Part of the Management for T2DM: from Animal Models to Human Clinical Studies. Curr Diab Rep. 2020;20(4):13.

4 Zouhal H, Saeidi A, Salhi A, et al. Exercise Training and Fasting: Current Insights. Open Access J Sports Med. 2020;11:1-28.

Chapter 4

1 Meczekalski, B, Katulski, K, Czyzyk, A, Podfigurna-Stopa, A, Maciejewska-Jeske, M. Functional hypothalamic amenorrhea and its influence on women's health. J Endocrinol Invest. 2014 Nov;37(11):1049-56. PMID: 25201001

2 Meczekalski, B, Podfigurna-Stopa, A, Warenik-Szymankiewicz A, Genazzani, AR. Functional hypothalamic amenorrhea: current view on neuroendocrine aberrations. Gynecol Endocrinol. 2008 Jan;24(1):4-11. PMID: 18224538

3 Martin, B, Pearson, M, Kebejian, L, Golden, E, Keselman A, Bender, M, Carlson, O, Egan, J, Ladenheim, B, Cadet, JL, Becker, KG, Wood, W, Duffy, K, Vinayakumar, P, Maudsley, S, Mattson, MP. Sex-dependent metabolic, neuroendocrine, and cognitive responses to dietary energy restriction and excess. Endocrinology. 2007 Sep;148(9):4318-33. PMID: 17569758

4 Kumar, S, Kaur, G. Intermittent fasting dietary restriction regimen negatively influences reproduction in young rats: a study of hypothalamo-hypophysial-gonadal axis. PLoS One. 2013;8(1):e52416. PMID: 23382817

5 Lopez-minguez J, Gómez-abellán P, Garaulet M. Timing of Breakfast, Lunch, and Dinner. Effects on Obesity and Metabolic Risk. Nutrients. 2019;11(11) PMID: 31684003

Chapter 5

1 Harvie M, Wright C, Pegington M, et al. The effect of intermittent energy and carbohydrate restriction v. daily energy restriction on weight loss and metabolic disease risk markers in overweight women. Br J Nutr. 2013;110(8):1534-47. PMID: 23591120

2 Dong TA, Sandesara PB, Dhindsa DS, et al. Intermittent Fasting: A Heart Healthy Dietary Pattern?. Am J Med. 2020; PMID: 32330491

3 Parvaresh A, Razavi R, Abbasi B, et al. Modified alternate-day fasting vs. calorie restriction in the treatment of patients with metabolic syndrome: A randomized clinical trial. Complement Ther Med. 2019;47:102187.

4 Lévesque S, Pol JG, Ferrere G, Galluzzi L, Zitvogel L, Kroemer G. Trial watch: dietary interventions for cancer therapy. Oncoimmunology. 2019;8(7):1591878.

5 Starkova J, Hermanova I, Hlozkova K, Hararova A, Trka J. Altered Metabolism of Leukemic Cells: New Therapeutic Opportunity. Int Rev Cell Mol Biol. 2018;336:93-147.

6 O'donnell MJ, Yusuf S, Mente A, et al. Urinary sodium and potassium excretion and risk of cardiovascular events. JAMA. 2011;306(20):2229-38.

7 Brandhorst S, Choi IY, Wei M, et al. A Periodic Diet that Mimics Fasting Promotes Multi-System Regeneration, Enhanced Cognitive Performance, and Healthspan. Cell Metab. 2015;22(1):86-99. PMID: 26094889

Chapter 6

1 Mu Q, Kirby J, Reilly CM, Luo XM. Leaky Gut As a Danger Signal for Autoimmune Diseases. Front Immunol. 2017;8:598.

2 Schunck M, Zague V, Dietary Supplementation with Specific Collagen Peptides Has a Body Mass Index-Dependent Beneficial Effect on Cellulite Morphology, 2015 Dec 1; 18(12): 1340-1348. PMID: 4685482
3 4. Proksch E, Segger D, et al., Oral supplementation of specific collagen peptides has beneficial effects on human skin physiology: a double-blind, placebo-controlled study, 2014; 27(1): 47-55. PMID: 23949208
4 Chlorophyll and Chlorophyllin, Oregon State Univ. Link here
5 Grandjean, P, Landrigan, P.J., Developmental neurotoxicity of industrial chemicals. The Lancet, 2006 November, Vol. 368, No. 9553, p.2167-2178.
6 Panahi Y, Darvishi B, Jowzi N, Beiraghdar F, Sahebkar A. Chlorella vulgaris: A Multifunctional Dietary Supplement with Diverse Medicinal Properties. Curr Pharm Des. 2016;22(2):164-73.
7 Finamore A, Palmery M, Bensehaila S, Peluso I. Antioxidant, Immunomodulating, and Microbial-Modulating Activities of the Sustainable and Ecofriendly . Oxid Med Cell Longev. 2017;2017:3247528.
8 Brandhorst S, Choi IY, Wei M, et al., A Periodic Diet that Mimics Fasting Promotes Multi-System Regeneration, Enhanced Cognitive Performance, and Healthspan. 2015 Jul; 22(1): 86-99.
9 Wei M, Brandhorst S, Shelehchi M, et al. Fasting-mimicking diet and markers/risk factors for aging, diabetes, cancer, and cardiovascular disease. Sci Transl Med. 2017;9(377)
10 Choi IY, Piccio L, Childress P, et al. A Diet Mimicking Fasting Promotes Regeneration and Reduces Autoimmunity and Multiple Sclerosis Symptoms. Cell Rep. 2016;15(10):2136-2146.
11 Rangan P, Choi I, Wei M, et al. Fasting-Mimicking Diet Modulates Microbiota and Promotes Intestinal Regeneration to Reduce Inflammatory Bowel Disease Pathology. Cell Rep. 2019;26(10):2704-2719.e6.
12 *The Longevity Diet*, Valter Longo, PhD, 2018.
13 Panebianco C, Potenza A, Pazienza V, Fasting and engineered diets as powerful tool in the medical practice: an old approach in the new era. 2017 Nov; 5(21): 429.
14 *Mehanna HM, Moledina J, Travis J. Refeeding syndrome: what it is, and how to prevent and treat it. BMJ. 2008; 336 (7659):1495-8.*

Chapter 7

1 Faris MA, Kacimi S, Al-Kurd RA, Fararjeh MA, Bustanji YK, Mohammad MK, Sale ML. Intermittent fasting during Ramadan attenuates proinflammatory cytokines and immune cells in healthy subjects. Nutr Res. 2012 Dec;32(12):947-55. PMID: 23244540
2 Vasconcelos AR, Yshii LM, Viel TA, et al. Intermittent fasting attenuates lipopolysaccharide-induced neuroinflammation and memory impairment. Journal of Neuroinflammation. 2-14;11:85
3 Aksungar FB, Topkaya AE, Akyildiz M. Interleukin-6, C-reactive protein and biochemical parameters during prolonged intermittent fasting. Ann Nutr Metab. PMID: 17374948
4 Antunes F, Erustes AG, Costa AJ, et al. Autophagy and intermittent fasting: the connection for cancer therapy?. Clinics (Sao Paulo). 2018;73(suppl 1):e814s.
5 Lanzi R, Luzi L, Caumo A, et al. Elevated insulin levels contribute to the reduced growth hormone (GH) response to GH-releasing hormone in obese subjects. Metab Clin Exp. 1999;48(9):1152-6. PMID: 10484056
6 Ji S, Guan R, Frank SJ, Messina JL. Insulin inhibits growth hormone signaling via the growth hormone receptor/JAK2/STAT5B pathway. J Biol Chem. 1999;274(19):13434-42. PMID: 10224108
7 Waugh DJ, Wilson C. The interleukin-8 pathway in cancer. Clin Cancer Res. 2008;14(21):6735-41. PMID: 18980965
8 Unalacak M, Kara IH, Baltaci D, Erdem O, Bucaktepe PG. Effects of Ramadan fasting on biochemical and hematological parameters and cytokines in healthy and obese individuals. Metab Syndr Relat Disord. 2011;9(2):157-61. PMID: 21235381
9 Schwartz L, Seyfried T, Alfarouk KO, Da veiga moreira J, Fais S. Out of Warburg effect: An effective cancer treatment targeting the tumor specific metabolism and dysregulated pH. Semin Cancer Biol. 2017;43:134-138.
10 Shackelford, D. B., & Shaw, R. J. (2009). The LKB1–AMPK pathway: metabolism and growth control in tumour suppression. *Nature Reviews Cancer*, *9*(8), 563–575. PMID: 19629071

11 Faubert, B., Boily, G., Izreig, S., Griss, T., Samborska, B., Dong, Z., ... Jones, R. G. (2013). AMPK is a negative regulator of the warburg effect and suppresses tumor growth in vivo. *Cell Metabolism*, *17*(1), 113–124. PMID: 23274086

12 Draznin, B., Wang, C., Adochio, R., Leitner, J. W., & Cornier, M. A. (2012). Effect of dietary macronutrient composition on AMPK and SIRT1 expression and activity in human skeletal muscle. *Hormone and Metabolic Research*, *44*(9), 650–655. PMID: 22674476

13 Cantó, C., Jiang, L. Q., Deshmukh, A. S., Mataki, C., Coste, A., Lagouge, M., ... Auwerx, J. (2010). Interdependence of AMPK and SIRT1 for Metabolic Adaptation to Fasting and Exercise in Skeletal Muscle. *Cell Metabolism*, *11*(3), 213–219. PMID: 20197054

14 Dogan, S., Johannsen, A. C., Grande, J. P., & Cleary, M. P. (2011). Effects of intermittent and chronic calorie restriction on mammalian target of rapamycin (mTOR) and IGF-I signaling pathways in mammary fat pad tissues and mammary tumors. *Nutrition and Cancer*, *63*(3), 389–401. PMID: 21462085

15 McDaniel, S. S., Rensing, N. R., Thio, L. L., Yamada, K. A., & Wong, M. (2011). The ketogenic diet inhibits the mammalian target of rapamycin (mTOR) pathway. *Epilepsia*, *52*(3). PMID: 21371020

16 De groot S, Pijl H, Van der hoeven JJM, Kroep JR. Effects of short-term fasting on cancer treatment. J Exp Clin Cancer Res. 2019;38(1):209.

17 Iyikesici MS. Survival outcomes of metabolically supported chemotherapy combined with ketogenic diet, hyperthermia, and hyperbaric oxygen therapy in advanced gastric cancer. Niger J Clin Pract. 2020;23(5):734-740.

18 Iyikesici MS. Long-Term Survival Outcomes of Metabolically Supported Chemotherapy with Gemcitabine-Based or FOLFIRINOX Regimen Combined with Ketogenic Diet, Hyperthermia, and Hyperbaric Oxygen Therapy in Metastatic Pancreatic Cancer. Complement Med Res. 2020;27(1):31-39.

19 Iyikesici MS. Feasibility study of metabolically supported chemotherapy with weekly carboplatin/paclitaxel combined with ketogenic diet, hyperthermia and hyperbaric oxygen therapy in metastatic non-small cell lung cancer. Int J Hyperthermia. 2019;36(1):446-455.

20 Seyfried TN, Yu G, Maroon JC, D'agostino DP. Press-pulse: a novel therapeutic strategy for the metabolic management of cancer. Nutr Metab (Lond). 2017;14:19.

21 Safdie FM, Dorff T, Quinn D, et al. Fasting and cancer treatment in humans: A case series report. Aging (Albany NY). 2009;1(12):988-1007. PMID: 20157582

22 Safdie FM, Dorff T, Quinn D, et al. Fasting and cancer treatment in humans: A case series report. Aging (Albany NY). 2009;1(12):988-1007.

23 Dorff TB, Groshen S, Garcia A, et al. Safety and feasibility of fasting in combination with platinum-based chemotherapy. BMC Cancer. 2016;16:360.

24 Bauersfeld SP, Kessler CS, Wischnewsky M, et al. The effects of short-term fasting on quality of life and tolerance to chemotherapy in patients with breast and ovarian cancer: a randomized cross-over pilot study. BMC Cancer. 2018;18(1):476.

25 NIDDK: NIH: Health Statistics – Digestive Diseases

26 Alonso S, Yilmaz ÖH. Nutritional Regulation of Intestinal Stem Cells. Annu Rev Nutr. 2018;38:273-301.

27 Mihaylova MM, Cheng CW, Cao AQ, Tripathi S, Mana MD, Bauer-Rowe KE, Abu-Remaileh M, Clavain L, Erdemir A, Lewis CA, Freinkman E, Dickey AS, La Spada AR, Huang Y, Bell GW, Deshpande V, Carmeliet P, Katajisto P, Sabatini DM, Yilmaz ÖH. Fasting Activates Fatty Acid Oxidation to Enhance Intestinal Stem Cell Function during Homeostasis and Aging. Cell Stem Cell. 2018 May 3;22(5):769-778.e4. doi: 10.1016/j.stem.2018.04.001. PMID: 29727683

28 Tavakkoli H, Haghdani S, Emami MH, Adilipour H, Tavakkoli M, Tavakkoli M. Ramadan fasting and inflammatory bowel disease. Indian J Gastroenterol. 2008;27(6):239-41.

29 Rangan P, Choi I, Wei M, et al. Fasting-Mimicking Diet Modulates Microbiota and Promotes Intestinal Regeneration to Reduce Inflammatory Bowel Disease Pathology. Cell Rep. 2019;26(10):2704-2719.e6.

30 Roy U., Gálvez E.J.C., Iljazovic A., Lesker T.R., Błażejewski A.J., Pils M.C., Heise U., Huber S., Flavell R.A., Strowig T. Distinct microbial communities trigger colitis development upon intestinal barrier damage via innate or adaptive immune cells. Cell Rep. 2017;21:994–1008.

31 Zhang X, Zou Q, Zhao B, et al. Effects of alternate-day fasting, time-restricted fasting and intermittent energy restriction DSS-induced on colitis and behavioral disorders. Redox Biol. 2020;32:101535.
32 Karakan T. Intermittent fasting and gut microbiota. Turk J Gastroenterol. 2019 Dec;30(12):1008. doi: 10.5152/tjg.2019.101219. PMID: 31854304
33 Mu Q, Kirby J, Reilly CM, Luo XM. Leaky Gut As a Danger Signal for Autoimmune Diseases. Front Immunol. 2017;8:598.
34 Blomberg J, Gottfries CG, Elfaitouri A, Rizwan M, Rosén A. Infection Elicited Autoimmunity and Myalgic Encephalomyelitis/Chronic Fatigue Syndrome: An Explanatory Model. Front Immunol. 2018;9:229.
35 Vojdani A, Pollard KM, Campbell AW. Environmental triggers and autoimmunity. Autoimmune Dis. 2014;2014:798029. doi: 10.1155/2014/798029. Epub 2014 Dec 24. PMID: 25610638
36 Leszek J, Trypka E, Tarasov VV, Ashraf GM, Aliev G. Type 3 Diabetes Mellitus: A Novel Implication of Alzheimers Disease. Curr Top Med Chem. 2017;17(12):1331-1335.
37 Vinciguerra F, Graziano M, Hagnäs M, Frittitta L, Tumminia A. Influence of the Mediterranean and Ketogenic Diets on Cognitive Status and Decline: A Narrative Review. Nutrients. 2020;12(4)
38 Van der Kooij MA, Fantin M, Rejmak E, Grosse J, Zanoletti O, Fournier C,Ganguly K,Kalita K, Kaczmarek L, Sandi C. Role for MMP-9 in stress-induced downregulation of nectin-3 in hippocampal CA1 and associated behavioural alterations. Nature Communications, 2014; 5: 4995.
39 Holth JK, Fritschi SK, Wang C, Pedersen NP, Cirrito JR, Mahan TE, Finn MB, Manis M, Geerling JC, Fuller PM, Lucey BP, Holtzman DM. The sleep-wake cycle regulates brain interstitial fluid tau in mice and CSF tau in humans. Science, 2019.
40 The sleep deprived brain. Dana Foundation. Link Here
41 Zhao Z, Zhao X, Veasey SC. Neural Consequences of Chronic Short Sleep: Reversible or Lasting? Front Neurol. 2017 May 31;8:235. doi: 10.3389/fneur.2017.00235. PMID: 28620347
42 Lucas G. Gut thinking: the gut microbiome and mental health beyond the head. Microb Ecol Health Dis. 2018 Nov 30;29(2):1548250. doi: 10.1080/16512235.2018.1548250. PMID: 30532687
43 Appleton J. The Gut-Brain Axis: Influence of Microbiota on Mood and Mental Health. Integr Med (Encinitas). 2018 Aug;17(4):28-32. PMID: 31043907
44 Rogers GB, Keating DJ, Young RL, Wong ML, Licinio J, Wesselingh S. From gut dysbiosis to altered brain function and mental illness: mechanisms and pathways. Mol Psychiatry. 2016 Jun;21(6):738-48. doi: 10.1038/mp.2016.50. Epub 2016 Apr 19. PMID: 27090305
45 Clapp M, Aurora N, Herrera L, Bhatia M, Wilen E, Wakefield S. Gut microbiota's effect on mental health: The gut-brain axis. Clin Pract. 2017 Sep 15;7(4):987. doi: 10.4081/cp.2017.987. PMID: 29071061
46 Brod M, Pohlman B, Højbjerre L, Adalsteinsson JE, Rasmussen MH. Impact of adult growth hormone deficiency on daily functioning and well-being. BMC Res Notes. 2014;7:813.
47 Baker LD, Barsness SM, Borson S, et al. Effects of growth hormone–releasing hormone on cognitive function in adults with mild cognitive impairment and healthy older adults: results of a controlled trial. Arch Neurol. 2012;69(11):1420-9.
48 Li L, Wang Z, Zuo Z. Chronic intermittent fasting improves brain cognitive functions and brain structures in mice. PLoS One. 2013 Jun 3;8(6):e66069. PMID: 23755298
49 Diniz BS, Teixeira AL. Brain-derived neurotrophic factor and Alzheimer's disease: physiopathology and beyond. Neuromolecular Med. 2011 Dec;13(4):217-22. PMID: 21898045
50 Baik SH, Rajeev V, Fann DY, Jo DG, Arumugam TV. Intermittent fasting increases adult hippocampal neurogenesis. Brain Behav. 2020;10(1):e01444.
51 Jamshed H, Beyl RA, Della manna DL, Yang ES, Ravussin E, Peterson CM. Early Time-Restricted Feeding Improves 24-Hour Glucose Levels and Affects Markers of the Circadian Clock, Aging, and Autophagy in Humans. Nutrients. 2019;11(6)
52 Shetty AK, Kodali M, Upadhya R, Madhu LN. Emerging Anti-Aging Strategies - Scientific Basis and Efficacy. Aging Dis. 2018;9(6):1165-1184.

Chapter 9

1 Meidenbauer JJ, Mukherjee P, Seyfried TN. The glucose ketone index calculator: a simple tool to monitor therapeutic efficacy for metabolic management of brain cancer. Nutr Metab (Lond). 2015; 12:12. Published 2015 Mar 11. PMCID: 4367849

Chapter 11

1 Mattson MP, Wan R. Beneficial effects of intermittent fasting and caloric restriction on the cardiovascular and cerebrovascular systems. J Nutr Biochem. 2005;16(3):129-37.

2 Ruiqian Wan, Simonetta Camandola, Mark P. Mattson, Intermittent Food Deprivation Improves Cardiovascular and Neuroendocrine Responses to Stress in Rats, *The Journal of Nutrition*, Volume 133, Issue 6, June 2003, Pages 1921–1929

3 Ohta S. Molecular hydrogen as a novel antioxidant: overview of the advantages of hydrogen for medical applications. *Methods Enzymol.* 2015; 555:289-317. PMID: 25747486

4 Hanaoka T, Kamimura N, Yokota T, Takai S, Ohta S. Molecular hydrogen protects chondrocytes from oxidative stress and indirectly alters gene expressions through reducing peroxynitrite derived from nitric oxide. *Med Gas Res.* 2011; 1(1): 18. Published 2011 Aug 4. PMCID: 3231990

5 Yokota T, Kamimura N, Igarashi T, Takahashi H, Ohta S, and Oharazawa H. Protective effect of molecular hydrogen against oxidative stress caused by peroxynitrite derived from nitric oxide in rat retina. *Clin Exp Ophthalmol.* 2015 Aug; 43(6): 568-77. PMID: 25801048

6 Slingerland AE, Schwabkey Z, Wiesnoski DH, Jenq RR. Clinical Evidence for the Microbiome in Inflammatory Diseases. *Front Immunol.* 2017; 8: 400. Published 2017 Apr 12. PMCID: 5388779

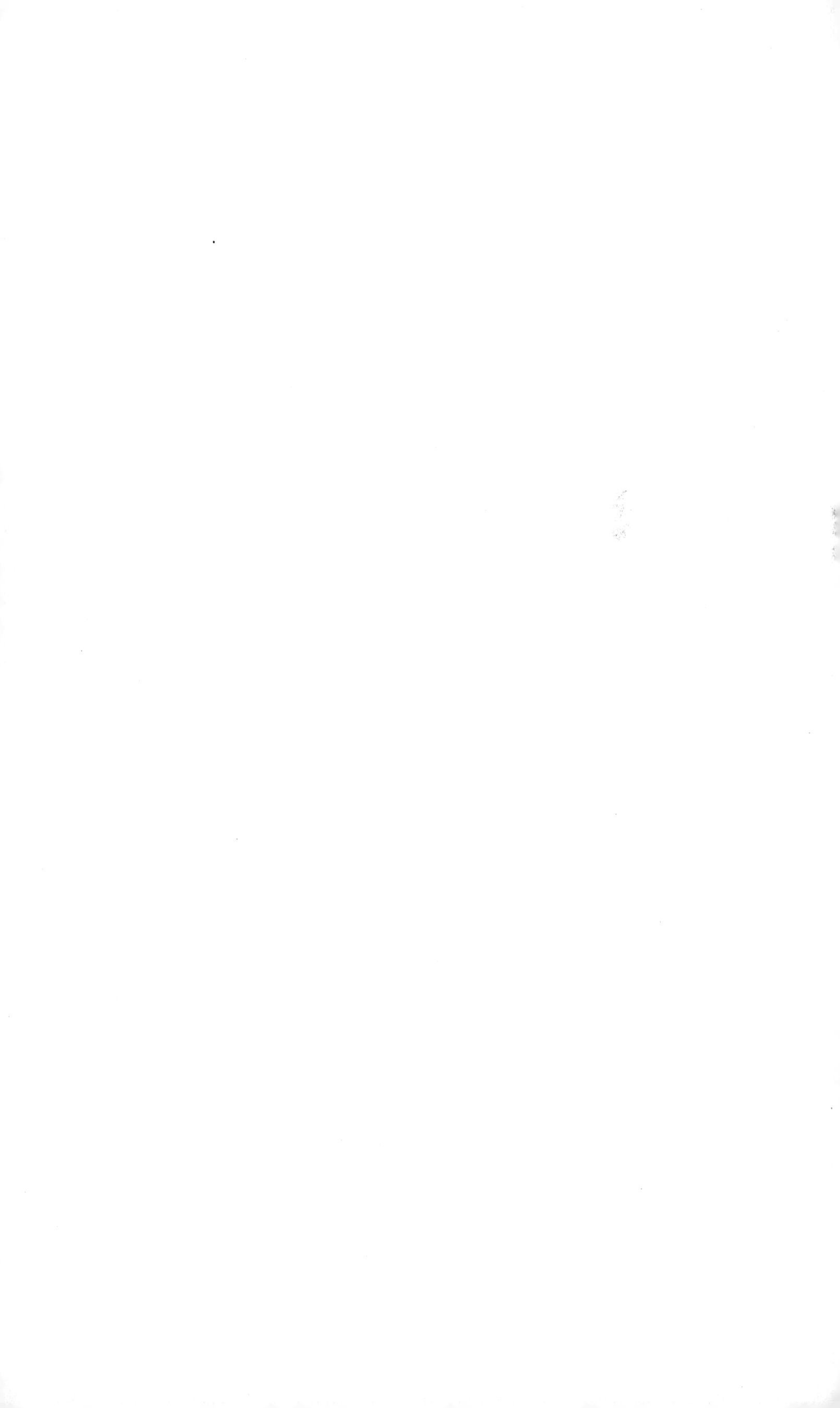

Printed in Great Britain
by Amazon